RESIDENTIAL VERSUS COMMUNITY CARE

Also by the author:

Women and Attempted Suicide
Empowerment in Community Care (editor)

RESIDENTIAL VERSUS COMMUNITY CARE

THE ROLE OF INSTITUTIONS IN WELFARE PROVISION

edited by

Dr Raymond Jack

MACMILLAN

First published 1998 by
MACMILLAN PRESS LTD
Houndmills, Basingstoke, Hampshire RG21 6XS
and London
Companies and representatives throughout the world

ISBN 0–333–66518–X paperback

A catalogue record for this book is available from the British Library.

This book is printed on paper suitable for recycling and
made from fully managed and sustained forest sources.

10 9 8 7 6 5 4 3 2 1
07 06 05 04 03 02 01 00 99 98

Editing and origination by
Aardvark Editorial, Mendham, Suffolk

Printed in Malaysia

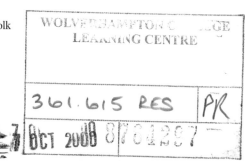

to my parents, Herbert and Beryl

CONTENTS

NOTES ON CONTRIBUTORS

Professor David Brandon is Professor of Community Care at Anglia Polytechnic University, Chelmsford. He was a social work practitioner, a Buddhist monk and, subsequently, Regional Director of MIND (The National Association for Mental Health) before becoming a teacher and researcher. He has been an influential advocate of community and user-led services, particularly for people with learning difficulties and mental health problems.

Richard Clough is General Secretary of the Social Care Association, an independent organisation which has long been an influential force in the development of policy and practice in residential care in Britain.

Professor Bleddyn Davies is Director of the Personal Social Services Research Unit at the University of Kent and the London School of Economics, which, for two decades, has been internationally influential in research in community care policy and practice.

Mervyn Eastman is Director of Social Services in the London Borough of Enfield. For many years, he was a practitioner and manager of services for older people, with a particular interest in elder abuse – conducting one of the earliest British studies of elder abuse and subsequently writing widely on the subject.

Dr Raymond Jack is Reader in Social Work at Anglia Polytechnic University, Chelmsford. Following 14 years of social work practice, he has been a teacher and researcher for ten years in various universities. He has written widely on community care policy and practice.

Professor Kathleen Jones is Emeritus Professor of Social Policy at the University of York. She has been researching the role of institutions in mental health in Britain, Europe and the USA for many years and has written extensively on the implementation of community care policy and practice in relation to people with psychiatric disorders.

Leonie Kellaher is a researcher at the Centre for Environmental and Social Studies in Ageing at the University of North London. She has written widely on the influence of environmental factors on the quality of care and the quality of life for residents of residential homes.

Jo Moriarty and **Enid Levin** are researchers for the National Institute for Social Work, London. They are both concerned with the long-term care of elderly and disabled people and the role of residential and community care services in maintaining them. They have recently completed and published a major study of respite care services.

Professor Sally Redfern is Director of the Nursing Research Unit at Kings College, London. She has a particular interest in the support of elderly people in long-stay settings and the future role of the nursing profession in residential and community care.

Yvonne Shemmings was, for many years, a social work practitioner and subsequently senior manager of elder care services for Essex County Council. She has recently completed and published a research study on death and dying in residential homes.

Dr Naom Trieman is Assistant Director and **Professor Julian Leff** is Honorary Director of the 'Team for the Assessment of Psychiatric Services' (TAPS) at the Institute of Psychiatry, London University, which for almost a decade has been researching the effects of mental hospital closure on patients and community care services in London.

INTRODUCTION

This book poses a challenge to a conventional wisdom that has emerged over the past 30 years amongst practitioners and policy makers in health and welfare, which at its most extreme asserts that residential care has 'no significant role to play in a modern welfare system' (Oliver, 1993, p. 13). The effect of this has been to relegate residential institutions to the status of an undesirable last resort on the margins of community care.

The contributions – common concerns and shared aspirations

The 12 chapters within the book deal with numerous types of residential institution ranging from monasteries to prisons, but they share a conviction that this conventional wisdom is ill-founded and that, on the contrary, such institutions do have a role in the production of welfare in communities. As such, they are integral to the process of community care and not a last ditch alternative to it.

The diverse contributions of our authors re-examine the origins of the policy and practice of institutional closure and community care. The critique of residential institutions by Goffman and Townsend – the 'literature of dysfunction' – is revisited, and it emerges that their conclusions in relation to the adverse effects of institutions were poorly supported by their evidence. There is ample reason to believe that the influence that these works have subsequently enjoyed has been more to do with political and professional pragmatism than with the scientific validity or practical utility of their findings, and the nature of the political and professional pressures that promoted the abandonment of publicly provided residential care as a legitimate form of intervention in health and welfare are disclosed. The past, present and future role of such provision in a variety of fields is examined against the background of community care policy and practice.

Chapter 1 provides the context for the contributions that follow. I briefly review the origins of the anti-residential care movement within the 'literature of dysfunction', which began to emerge in the late 1950s and generally offered an alarming indictment of conditions and practices in mental hospitals, old people's homes and other residential institutions. This critique has had a profound negative impact on professional and public attitudes towards residential institutions and the subsequent development of community care policy and practice. However, there is reason to believe that this impact has been due more to eloquent rhetoric than scientific reason, that the critique has been conceptually flawed and that much of the research on which it is based is methodologically inadequate. This has contributed not only to the flight from the public provision of residential care, but also to a damaging misconception of how welfare is produced in communities – how communities care – which ignores the interdependence of all the 'institutions' involved in its production, not least the family and other sources of care in our society. New models are needed which avoid the naïve dualism of 'residential care is bad, community care is good' and which, by developing a more systemic understanding of the process of community care, will enable us fully to integrate residential institutions into this process rather than marginalise them, to the detriment of their residents, carers and the wider communities they serve.

The next four chapters develop the theme of the interdependence of institutions in community care by considering three very different types of residential institution – mental hospitals, prisons, and old people's homes and monasteries. What emerges is a picture not only of the continuing need for these institutions, but also of their permeability, as opposed to the isolation conventionally attributed to them as archetypal 'total institutions'.

Chapter 2 by Dr Naom Trieman and Professor Julian Leff is an up-to-the-minute account of a major study of psychiatric hospital closure that has been carried out over the past decade in London. The closure of two large, old mental hospitals in the capital provided a unique opportunity to assess the impact of an ambitious attempt to replace psychiatric care in institutions entirely with community-based provision. The study is of particular relevance to our collection of readings as it specifically studied the impact of hospital closure on other services in the area, patients, relatives, staff and the wider community, in other words on the production of welfare within the whole community. The findings that continue to emerge from this sophisticated enquiry are challenging to the conventional wisdom of decarceration because, whilst evidence clearly emerged that the majority of ex-long-stay patients benefited from moving into the community, many did not, and serious problems have emerged in other areas of the care system. These problems include a 'crisis situation' in relation to acute admission and rehabilitation. The authors conclude that a relatively small proportion of chronically ill patients will 'always need some sort of long term inpatient care' and that 'for the residual group of severely disabled patients... adequate care in community facilities is not possible'.

Chapter 3, by Greg Mantle – a practising probation officer, lecturer and researcher – offers further insights into the interdependence of residential and other institutions in his discussion of the role of prisons in our communities. For many, prison is the archetypal total institution perceived within this conceptual framework as being deliberately designed to achieve the impermeability and segregation said to be definitive characteristics of such institutions. Early in his chapter, however, he points to the similarities between the captivity imposed by incarceration in these institutions and that imposed by poverty and other institutionalised disadvantage experienced in the community by prisoners and ex-prisoners. He argues that prisons are the product of the communities they exist within and serve social purposes beyond the merely punitive; as such, no valid critique can consider them as being separate from wider criminal justice policy and practice or indeed the wider social processes that produce both custody and its alternatives.

In Chapter 4, Professor Bleddyn Davies – who for two decades has been in the forefront of community care policy formulation – considers the development of a 'new species' of long-term shelter-with-care. The discussion challenges the assumption that community care policy and practice is an alternative to residential care; rather, Professor Davies shows how the community care reforms in the UK provide opportunities for the evolution of new forms of such care. However, a lack of vision – I would suggest due in part to the conventional wisdom of anti-residential care – is seen as leading to slow change and an 'over ready acceptance of virtually traditional forms of provision'. Examples are given from America of 'horizon broadening developments' in forms of shelter-with-care that share the common characteristic of blurring the boundaries between home care and residential care. In this sense, the discussion gives very practical examples of the interdependence and permeability of the various types of institution involved in the provision of community care.

Chapter 5, by Professor David Brandon – a long-standing advocate of community care, particularly for people with learning difficulties –

continues to develop this theme of the interdependence of institutions in community care. Professor Brandon interprets the monastic tradition as the beginning of community care rather than its antithesis. Drawing on historical data, he compares the Western monastic tradition with Buddhist monasticism. Christian monasticism in the Middle Ages is seen as inward looking and as turning away from the world (renunciation), which is contrasted with the Buddhist tradition of community service. Whilst the Buddhist monastery undeniably meets some of the criteria of Goffman's 'total institution', there are links with the outside world such that the ethic of the Buddhist monk is that of serving the practical needs of the world rather than withdrawing from it. Within the monastic walls, the 'disease of individualism' could be effectively countered, but meeting the needs of the sick and poor outside the walls was equally important. There was much exchange: monks came and went voluntarily without a sense of failure at leaving or re-entering, local residents came in for meditation and advice, and there was medical assistance. The theme, not of separation from the community but of interaction with it, is revisited several times and in different ways to demonstrate the potential for residential institutions to be a genuine part of the process of community care.

Chapter 5 focuses on one specific function of residential homes – respite care for elderly people. It draws extensively on research from around the world relating to residential care policy and practice and offers evidence-based conclusions on the role of good quality residential provision in community care.

Jo Moriarty and Enid Levin, from the National Institute for Social Work, have spent 10 years researching the ways in which communities care for frail elderly and disabled people. In Chapter 6, they describe their research into various forms of respite care and the relationship between residential respite care, other forms of respite and other services. Whilst focusing on care for older people, they refer to evidence from many nations and relating to various client groups. They explore the proposition that residential respite care is indispensable to the continued functioning of community-based services. They suggest that conventional assumptions about the role of residential care in general have 'muddied the waters' and prevented the full potential of this form of care being realised.

Anyone reading the next three chapters will, at the very least, be required to reconsider the assertion that there is no place in a civilised society for residential institutions. On the contrary, these authors share a conviction that the provision of high-quality, publicly funded residential care for the chronically sick and dying is a measure of how civilised a society is.

In Chapter 7, Professor Kathleen Jones – an eminent critic of inadequate community care policy and practice in relation to mentally ill people – turns her attention to the abandonment of chronically sick and elderly people by the National Health Service (NHS) since the advent of community care and the mixed economy of care. As Professor Jones wryly observes, 'people do not die to schedule', and this poses problems within the contract culture imposed by the National Health Service and Community Care Act 1990. Through the sensitive use of case studies and policy analysis, a damning indictment unfolds of the callous neglect of disabled and dying people who are now routinely denied care in hospitals that no longer possess long-term care beds. Helpless patients are being thrust out into the community to be 'cared' for by fragmented and inadequate services, which, Professor Jones concludes, will never be able to provide appropriate tending for people who need continuous nursing care. Several practical proposals for improving this dire situation are offered.

The theme of the indispensable – and apparently growing – role of residential care for many dying people is developed from a different perspective by Yvonne Shemmings, who for several years was a senior manager of elder care services for a large shire county. Chapter 8 is a description of the findings of Yvonne's research into the effects of caring for dying people on care assistants in old people's homes. Again, there is a telling interweaving of policy analysis and at times very moving case studies, which illustrate the stress endured by these workers who 'experience more loss in six months than most of us feel in a lifetime'. The prolonged devaluation of residential care and of the skills involved in providing it has left staff ill-trained and ill-prepared for the daunting task they face. The chapter concludes with suggestions for remedying this enduring neglect.

Kathleen Jones and Yvonne Shemmings both suggest that, far from further reductions in publicly provided residential care for chronically sick and dying people, more places are required in hospitals and residential homes and that the quality of care within them needs to meet the highest professional standards.

In Chapter 9, Professor Sally Redfern of the Nursing Research Unit, Kings College, London examines the implications for the development of the nursing profession of the new managerialism and contract culture resulting from the community care legislation. Professor Redfern is concerned that, under the financial and other pressures of the mixed economy, there may be a process of deprofessionalisation afoot. Euphemistically referred to as 'multiskilling' and 'skill mix', the skills of basic nursing care are, in the interests of parsimony, said to be no longer the preserve of the trained nurse but may be practised instead by less expensive support staff, including porters and clerical workers. With the abandonment of continuing care in favour of high-tech acute care within the NHS, two questions remain unanswered – what will be the future for the holistic approach to patients' needs, which is a central element of the nursing profession, and, in its absence, who will provide the skilled care needed by hundreds of thousands of chronically sick, disabled and dying people?

Chapters 10 and 11 continue the discussion of standards of practice in residential care, but from different perspectives.

Chapter 10 draws extensively on international research in a discussion of the nature of quality in residential care, and how it can be assessed and promoted. Leonie Kellaher is a researcher at the Centre for Environmental and Social Studies in Ageing, which for many years has been a prolific and influential source of research and evidence-based policy and practice guidance. The focus is on the need for residential homes to support individuals in maintaining their sense of self-hood, which the total institution threatens. However, Leonie asserts that conventional views of the residential institution as inevitably depersonalising are based on an 'overgrowth of domestic and familial analogy', which bear little relationship to the current realities of collective living. We require new perspectives on homes, which need to be seen no longer as 'monolithic' but as permeable and intimately connected to their communities The chapter offers guidance on best practice derived from the findings of the Caring in Homes initiative, which was a practice-based research project designed to identify and promote those elements in residential practice that support the resident in their defence of the self.

Mervyn Eastman is a Director of Social Services in London who for 25 years has practised in and managed services for older people. He has written extensively on elder abuse and in Chapter 11 brings the two elements of his experience together in a discussion of how it is that abuse of all forms still persists in homes and what the role of managers is in both its perpetuation and its prevention. Mervyn explores the nexus between managers, care workers and residents, and discusses how care can be 'corrupted' within this. The answers he proposes, in his own words, lie somewhere between total management incompetence and blatant collusion based on a potentially fatal combination of ageism, fear, ignorance and denial. Within this nexus, individual residents are marginalised or discounted. Practice guidance is offered on how these 'blockages' can be confronted, based on the acceptance by managers of their own individual responsibility and personal vision of the integrity and worth of each individual resident. The conclusion is that, in abusive situations, not only are the residents 'sans everything', but so too are the ineffective managers of what should have been the victims' homes.

The various contributions to this book clearly demonstrate the conviction of their authors that there will always be a need for high-quality residential provision in caring communities, a conviction based on many years of professional and personal experience in health and welfare practice, research and policy formulation. The final chapter is no exception.

Richard Clough has spent a professional career working in residential institutions and trying to promote high-quality residential care, a contribution recognised in the conferment of the OBE. He is currently the Chief Executive of the Social Care Association, which for many years was known as the Residential Care Association, a change of title which signifies his belief that residential provision is an indispensable part of social care within our community. In Chapter 12, Richard offers a personal view of the damaging effects of the perennial devaluation of residential care amongst health and welfare professionals and the impact of the new community care on this care sector. Undaunted, however, by this history of criticism and neglect, he gives a balanced appraisal of the dangers and opportunities of collective living for various consumer groups. He concludes with an optimistic view of how many aspects of the community care legislation can promote high-quality residential care, which will provide a rewarding experience for both those who provide it and those who reside within it.

The context – the crisis in community care

In the rush to implement 'community care' in health and welfare, assumptions about the limited worth and even more limited future of care in residential institutions have gone largely unchallenged. This has resulted in the wholesale abandonment of residential provision in the public sector of health and welfare, a situation which already threatens to undermine the provision of a continuum of care both in the community and within the institutional residential care sector. There is currently a 100 per cent plus occupancy rate of psychiatric beds in the UK, which clearly stems from the massive reduction in such provision that has occurred in the past 20 years. In 1976,

97,000 beds were available for mental illness admissions, this having reduced to 55,000 by 1991, whilst during the same period the number of admissions increased from 179,000 to 219,000 (Jones, 1993, p. 244).

The closure of local authority homes for old people has similarly placed strains on the health service in terms of maintaining throughput in general hospital beds. Between 1983 and 1993 the number of people aged 85 and over in England increased from 541,000 to 840,000, whilst the number of NHS geriatric beds available daily diminished from 56,000 to 38,000 and the number of places available in local authority homes for elderly people declined from 116,400 to 68,900 (Department of Health, 1995, pp. 11, 39 and 80).

The loss of institutional residential provision for other groups has received less public attention, although concern has recently been mounting in social services departments in Britain about the lack of suitable residential provision for children who – by dint of behavioural or other severe problems – are difficult to maintain in foster care (Valios, 1994, p. 6).

In July 1996 it was disclosed in the *Independent* that, earlier in the year, Prime Minister John Major had written a private letter to the Secretary of State for Health expressing serious concern over the policy of community care for mentally ill people and in particular the programme of closure of mental hospitals, which he asserted 'may have gone too far', such that there were now too few beds available for those who required 24 hour care and 'genuine asylum'. Reports from the Royal College of Psychiatrists suggest that bed occupancy rates are running at over 100 per cent 'with the beds of patients out on leave immediately filled by others' (Timmins, 1996, p. 1). The letter referred to the growing public anxiety over the perceived threat posed by mentally disordered patients being discharged to inadequate community care services and subsequently either engaging in acts of serious self-harm or committing murder – several highly publicised cases of self-injury and murder by patients recently discharged to community care having led to 'a growing public fear of the mentally ill'. The disclosure of this letter may well prove to be a milestone in the increasingly contentious history of community care in the UK and the role of residential institutions within it.

As doubts about the practicality of community care policies have mounted – particularly for people with mental illness in Britain, the USA and Italy, where sweeping policies of hospital closure predated the British experience – we are witnessing a revisionist backlash with demands for 're-institutionalisation'. A particularly sinister example is the inclusion in the American Republican party's manifesto of proposals for a reduction in community child care and a return to institutional provision in orphanages (Rhodes, 1994, p. 16). This is acknowledged by its proponents as a response to the allegedly unsustainable cost of social security payments to families in the community and, as such, has striking resemblance to the pressures that led to the reduction of 'outdoor relief' and the establishment of workhouses in Britain under the 1834 Poor Law Amendment Act. A reassessment of the proper role of institutions in community care is urgently needed to avoid a similar ominous and ill-advised flight back to the future in European social care.

References

Department of Health (1995) *Health and Personal Social Statistics for England.* London, HMSO.

Jones, K. (1993) *Asylums and After: A Revised History of the Mental Health Servies: From the Early 18th Century to the 1990s.* London, Athlone Press.

Oliver, M. (1993) Struggling for independence. *Community Care,* 2 September: 13.

Rhodes, T. (1994) Orphanages plan puts boys town in the limelight. *Times* 8 December: 16.

Timmins, N. (1996) *Independent,* 16 July:1.

Valios, N. (1994) Child residential bed shortage crisis looms. *Community Care,* 1–7 December: 6.

1 INSTITUTIONS IN COMMUNITY CARE

Raymond Jack

This chapter sets the context of the debate over the place of residential care within community care. It describes the anti-institutional rationale of the past three decades from Erving Goffman in the early 1960s, with his devastating critique of mental hospitals, to Michael Oliver's equally powerful indictment of the inadequacy of the residential response to people with disabilities in the 1990s. Whilst acknowledging the eloquence and perceptiveness of this 'literature of dysfunction' in relation to residential care, the methodological and conceptual inadequacy of such a 'dualistic' conception – 'residential care is bad, community care is good' – is described and discussed. An alternative, 'systemic' view of residential care within caring communities is developed, and, on the basis of the past 30 years' experience of alternative provision and recent research, the conclusion is drawn that residential institutions are an integral part of how communities care and that there will always be a place for this form of care in a civilised society.

Definitions and meanings

The word 'institution' is not easily understood as it is used to define a number of apparently highly dissimilar things – the *Concise English Dictionary*, for example, includes in its definition of institution 'Society or organisation for promotion of scientific, educational, or other public object' (Oxford University Press, 1979, p. 560). The Church is given as an example of such an organisation, and, whilst not being 'organisations' in this sense, the law and the family are commonly referred to as institutions (see Jones and Fowles, 1984, pp. 206–7 for a fuller discus-

10

sion of definitions). The dictionary then goes on to add that the word can be used to describe the 'building used by this (society or organisation)'. However, it becomes clear that an institution consists of something more than just bricks and mortar: there is something here which alludes to worthy purpose and social contribution – to process as well as structure and function. Another aspect of its meaning is described as 'Established law, custom or practice'; again, social process is emphasised as opposed to physical structure – an institution can exist without any associated physical structure. What is not included in the dictionary definition is any suggestion that the term 'institution' has pejorative meaning.

In this chapter, I want to suggest that, within the field of health and welfare policy and practice, which is our primary concern, the term 'institution' has been too narrowly understood, with consequences that go well beyond the semantic. It has become almost axiomatic that institutions are buildings – mental hospitals, children's homes, prisons and so on. Because this form of service provision – which may be broadly defined as 'residential' – has come to be viewed as undesirable for a variety of reasons we shall explore later, the social processes that go on within them are also viewed as *inevitably* undesirable. The term 'institutionalisation' describes these undesirable processes and briefly put involves symptoms, including apathy, withdrawal, loss of motivation and helplessness – all said to result from depersonalisation caused by block treatment in groups, routinisation and role deprivation. This has come to be inextricably associated with residential provision, and it is rarely acknowledged by the critics of residential care that other forms of service provision, usually described as 'community care' (domiciliary and day care, counselling and care management), may be viewed as institutions or that they may display similarly undesirable institutional processes.

Dualistic and systemic concepts of community care

This narrow conception of institutions and institutionalisation has constrained our understanding of the wider processes of health and welfare in communities. Until comparatively recently, 'informal carers' – family, neighbours and friends – had been neglected in the planning and provision of health and welfare services. Similarly, service users and providers have been perceived as somehow different species with little commonality of goals, skills, aspirations, with the inevitable professional paternalism that this entails. These are forms of dualistic thinking about the nature of caring in communities. In the same way, a dualistic view of residential and community care has arisen which perceives residential care as 'bad' and community care as 'good'. In this view, the so-called 'continuum of care' has an assumption underlying it of a progression from first choice to last resort that has damaging consequences for service users and providers alike. A set of intransigent, negative attitudes towards residential provision has been noted in a series of official reports and reviews of the literature (Barclay, 1982; Sinclair, 1988; Wagner, 1988). In 1981 a Department of Health study of community care noted a tendency to underestimate the numbers needing long-term care in institutions (Department of Health, 1981), and a year later the Barclay enquiry into the role and tasks of social work reported that the stigma attached to residential care was 'partly [to do] with the attitudes of those social workers and others who regard residential care as the [undesirable] last resort... the saying "a bad home is better than a good institution" still has its adherents' (Barclay, 1982, p. 57).

Alternatively, if we accept that the 'community' consists of a variety of institutions – including the family as well as a variety of caring services – a systemic view can emerge which conceives of an integrated network of institutions that are interdependent and complementary, rather than more and less desirable or just plain good and bad. This enables an understanding of the way in which the balance of care shifts in communities, not just between the formally designated caring services but between all the institutions within which care is provided. As the capability of the family to maintain and care for its 'dependants' changes, and cultural – popular and professional – expectations and interpretations of health and welfare provision shift, a systemic view enables a response to the needs of communities and individuals to emerge that is rooted in a more realistic understanding of wider social process.

In a systemic view, 'institutions' does not just mean residential facilities for 'dependent' people, nor does it entail assumptions about the comparative worth of one or another source of care provision. In the following discussion, I want to argue that the dualistic and largely pejorative view of residential institutional provision that has emerged over the past half century has not only been ill-informed, but has also been part of a wider misconception of the process of how communities care, which is having damaging results for individuals and for the communities on which we all depend for the satisfaction of our many and diverse needs. Central to this argument for a more systemic view of how communities care is the role of publicly provided residential care

in the production of social welfare, which I suggest cannot be fulfilled adequately by independent provision for several reasons:
First, there is a need for central planning of the production of welfare in communities. This does not necessarily mean a top-down, bureaucratic and paternalistic approach. It can be locally based and needs led.

One example is that of the Birmingham Community Care Special Action Project described by Wistow and Barnes, who give a convincing account of user involvement in community care planning and implementation (Wistow and Barnes, 1993).

At present, we have a situation in which the bulk of residential provision for older people is provided by the private and voluntary sector; welfare planning within this market-driven scenario is simply impossible: one dramatic change in interest rates or property market values can alter the dynamics of this type of private social care market. Independent sector providers have neither the incentive nor the information on which to make such long-term plans for the welfare of the community of which they legitimately only serve a very circumscribed market-driven need. Why should they devote resources to invest in such activity?

Second, the establishment of local authority social services departments in 1970 was designed to promote the integrated planning and provision of services to defined local communities. They were intended to promote the integration of services from a variety of different sectors of formal and informal, voluntary and private welfare – residential, domiciliary, social work and so on. (For a discussion of how this may be approached, see Henderson and Armstrong, 1993.) This is not possible in the absence of central planning and provision.

Third, the alleged benefits of competition between providers of, and commercialisation within, public services has been a driving force behind the ideology of a mixed economy of welfare. There will be problems if there is no publicly provided residential care to enable competition for a private sector inclined to merger and marginalisation of the small provider. Cost control will thus become increasingly difficult as public provision is diminished in a market of increasing need – as with the growing population of very elderly people. A recent review of monetarist government policy in relation to public expenditure on health and welfare from two eminent Oxford economists, published in the *National Institute Economic Review*, suggests that the commercialisation of public services will generally drive costs up and, far from reducing public expenditure, may well increase it. In addition, introducing commercial criteria into the management of public services is extremely difficult because the outputs are not as easy to measure as is productivity in other fields, such as running super-market chains (Flemming and Oppenheimer, 1996).

Fourth, the provision of a 'social wage' in the form of publicly provided welfare is an important source of social integration in a society as severely divided between the rich minority and poor majority as that of the UK. The commitment of the mass of people in compara-tive poverty to a social system dominated by a massively rich minority can only be sustained by such provision of a social wage that guaran-tees care from cradle to grave – this cannot be guaranteed without public provision. This applies not only to the poor, but also to the aspi-rant middle class, who – if they have no requirement to provide for the less fortunate, and receive increasingly poor public services for them-selves – will gradually withdraw behind security fences and private health and welfare provision, thereby heightening social divisions.

Fifth, social integration may well also be fostered by the very tangible social assets of residential provision – bricks and mortar in the form of hospitals and residential homes in communities for their 'dependent' members.

Sixth, there is doubt over the ability of older people especially to pay for privately provided care. The current generation of old people has been enabled to do so only as a result of capital accumulated through the property boom in the 1970s, which is unlikely to recur. Their children will be unable to inherit their wealth to pay for care if the parents have already exhausted their capital in paying for their own long-term care. This will directly affect not only the social care market for the next generation, but also the property market upon which so many other sectors of the economy depend. The danger of pauperisation for elderly people within the market for long-term social care is described by Bleddyn Davies (1990), and government recognition of this has led to recent – but unfortunately belated and inadequate – changes in the social security rules governing means testing in relation to residential care costs for older people. These changes increase the amount of capital people are allowed to retain; however, at £16,000 this will clearly be insufficient to make any real impact on the situation.

Finally, the abandonment of public residential provision has been in part justified by government pronouncements on the threat to national prosperity due to the allegedly unaffordable escalation of public expen-diture and consequent taxation resulting from what one government report described as a 'rising tide' of elderly infirm people. The threat-ened effects of what Margaret Thatcher once called the demographic time-bomb have been convincingly rejected by recent analysis (Falkingham, 1989) showing that the population of those over 65 and needing care is unlikely to increase significantly before the year 2020, a conclusion reinforced in a report from the all party Commons Health Committee in August 1996. This report asserted, after considering the available evidence, both that the age time-bomb is an alarmist myth with which government has colluded in order to promote its policies on public expenditure and taxation, and that 'continuing to fund long term care mainly from general taxation was a defensible option which is both possible and affordable' (Webster, 1996, p. 2).

For these reasons, therefore, the focus of this chapter will remain on public provision.

The rise and fall of 'institutions'

The second half of the 20th century has seen the rise and fall of confidence in social welfare as the solution to social problems – and for the past two decades welfare has been increasingly defined as part of the problem rather than the solution. This has not only been driven by the political ideology of the new right (McCarthy, 1989) but has also been fuelled by a loss of confidence within the social welfare professions over their role and tasks (Barclay, 1982). Perhaps the most dramatic manifestation of this has been the rejection of residential care as a legitimate care option for any client group. This followed more than a century of investment in institutional provision (Parker, 1988a), which saw not only a continuous growth in the numbers of children and adults being cared for in residential facilities, but also a gradual development of research-based theory and method, which transformed the physical and practice environment within the best residential care and began to address its interdependence with the wider community (Booth, 1985; Willcocks et al., 1987; Sinclair, 1988; Elkan and Kelly, 1991; National Institute for Social Work, 1993a).

By the early 1970s the burden of the workhouse – concisely described by Parker when he asserted 'the history of institutions in this country has been dominated by destitution, madness and criminality' (Parker, 1988a, p. 8) – was beginning to be dissipated. This was powered not only by the growth of professional knowledge and practice skill, but also through the comparative financial freedom bestowed by the economic growth of the 1960s – which enabled new investment in the residential stock – and the powerful vehicle for focused reform created with the establishment of the unified social services departments in 1970. For the first time, it became possible to conceive of residential care as part of an integrated approach to the planning and provision of social welfare to local communities; residential provision was to be conceived of as 'community homes' rather than as a stigmatising response to individual inadequacy or indigence (Seebohm, 1968).

The renaissance of residential provision was, however, to be short lived. The recurrent crises in the British economy beginning in the mid-1970s made the ambitious growth targets of 10 per cent per annum originally set for social services departments increasingly unattainable. Although recent analysis suggests that expenditure on the welfare state has at least been maintained over the past two decades (Hills, 1990), there is no doubt that there has been a collapse in the confidence of health and welfare professions in their ability to provide ever-improving services to increasing numbers of elderly, sick and disabled people. In this increasingly hostile financial environment and with the loss of confidence politically and professionally in the welfare solution, the commitment to provide publicly funded residential care began to be eroded.

Local authority residential provision was felt to consume a disproportionate amount of social service departments' budgets whilst serving only a minority of their clientele. The Audit Commission report *Managing Social Services for the Elderly More Effectively* (Audit Commission, 1985) found that only 2 per cent of elderly clients of social services departments were in residential care but that they consumed 55 per cent of the spending on this client group. Whether or not this was a legitimate distribution of expenditure, and whether alternative forms of provision for similarly disabled people are more cost-effective, this fact alone made this element of the continuum of care vulnerable. Sir Roy Griffiths' (1988) report on community care focused upon the apparent cost-ineffectiveness of residential care, comparing it with the apparent cost-effectiveness of community care. The National Health Service and Community Care Act 1990, based upon the Griffiths report – through its financial sanctions on local authorities providing their own residential care, for which they receive no community care funds – ensured the rapid reduction in public sector residential care that has since occurred through the closure or sale of many residential facilities to the independent sector. Demographic change, financial pressures and the government's radical response to them have converged to create a situation in which the remaining years of the century are witnessing what may be the last chance for public residential provision, which has for 150 years been the last refuge for the majority of people unable to afford private care.

This process of asset stripping of capital previously accumulated in public provision has been described as a self-inflicted wound and certainly represents a haemorrhage of social wealth, yet it has gone virtually unchallenged by professionals within health and welfare services who have, for the past three decades, revered the policy of community care and reviled the practice of residential provision. There is ample evidence to suggest, however, that this apparently eager compliance has been fundamentally misguided and owes more to rhetoric than to reason.

The literature of dysfunction

The literature of dysfunction consists of a series of influential publications, beginning in Britain with Russell Barton's monograph *Institutional Neurosis* (1959), in which this psychiatrist described what he perceived as the adverse effects for some patients of care in psychiatric hospitals. Peter Townsend's *The Last Refuge* (1962) detailed the allegedly detrimental effects of institutional care upon elderly people in late 1950s, concluding that this form of care should be phased out and rapidly replaced by sheltered housing units. Subsequently, a library of works similarly damning of residential care for various groups has been constructed, including Robb's *Sans Everything* (1967), describing the plight of geriatric patients, *Taken for a Ride* (1972), Michael Meacher's account of homes for elderly mentally ill people, and Clough's *Old Age Homes* (1981), whilst Miller and Gwynne (1972) deal with people with physical disability, and Morris (1969) provides a similarly unfavourable critique of residential provision for people with learning difficulties.

Perhaps the most influential book of this genre relating to mental health care has been Erving Goffman's *Asylums: Essays on the Social Situation of Mental Patients and Other Inmates* (1961), which constructed the concept of the 'total institution' and described the processes of depersonalisation and institutionalisation entailed in being a patient/resident within one. In relation to child care, John Bowlby's work on 'maternal deprivation', published over three decades between 1951 and 1980, described the damaging effects of breaking natural bonds between mother and child and raised fears about the possible adverse effects of residential care for children, thereby increasing professional disquiet about any form of residential provision (Bowlby, 1969).

This critique of residential care has been assimilated into the professional culture, becoming a 'conventional wisdom' and being regarded as self-evident truth. However, the alleged truth described in the literature of dysfunction is far from self-evident when subjected to closer scrutiny.

'Institutionalisation' reassessed

When considering the effects on individuals of living in residential institutions, any analysis that fails to take account of personality, life experience and social process before entry to the institution must be regarded with suspicion. Goffman's interest in asylums was but a part of his wider concern with the creation of social identity, and institutionalisation was considered to be part of this wider social process. Unfortunately – partly due to the nature of the situation he described in a particularly unprogressive state mental hospital – the wider analysis has been largely ignored in the subsequent discourse on institutions in favour of a narrow focus on residential institutions in isolation from this social context and process. The conventional wisdom resulting from this tunnel vision, which holds that all residential care results in institutionalisation and that this does not occur elsewhere in the community, is thus conceptually inadequate. In addition, there are methodological inadequacies in this body of research which undermine the credibility of the widely accepted claims of the critique of residential care.

Patients and residents are involved in social processes that promote their welfare to a greater or lesser extent before entering residential institutions. The neglect of this in much of the literature of dysfunction is a reflection of the dualistic conception of institutional care, which sees it as somehow separate from wider social process rather than as a product of it – a shortcoming that a more systemic analysis avoids. Such analysis, however, would require, for example, comparative and longitudinal methodologies that are absent from much of the critique of residential care, not least from the two most influential studies of Townsend and Goffman. Where longitudinal and comparative approaches have been employed, the findings cast doubt on the widely accepted claims about the adverse effects of institutional life for such residents. For example, in relation to the effects of institutionalisation on elderly residents of nursing homes, Tobin and Lieberman's study *Last Home for the Aged* found that the alleged adverse effects of institutional practices were actually present before the residents' entry to the home and stemmed from the circumstances surrounding their decision to enter it – such as family breakdown, abandonment and loss – rather than from entering the home (Tobin and Lieberman, 1976).

Similar conclusions were reached more recently by Willcocks and her colleagues, who studied 1,000 residents of old people's homes and whose approach regarded the dependency they found among these residents to be a continuation of processes already begun in the community (Willcocks et al., 1987).

In a similar vein, a comparative study of schizophrenics comparing the extent to which the proposed features of 'institutionalisation' were present in schizophrenics who had not received long-term hospital care with those who had found that:

> there was no difference between the two groups... the deficits of chronic schizophrenia are an integral feature of the disease process, and that any effects of institutionalisation are relatively small. (Johnstone et al., 1981, p. 195)

These conclusions are remarkably similar to an assertion of Russell Barton's, which is rarely acknowledged in the literature of dysfunction, that 'The condition [institutional neurosis] may be indistinguishable from the later stages of schizophrenia' and – perhaps of more concern – that 'None of the elements I will describe seems peculiar to total institutions' (Barton, 1959, pp. 13 and 15).

More recently, a large-scale study of de-institutionalisation has compared those patients left behind in a large London mental hospital with those discharged to 'community care'. The TAPS (The Team for the Assessment of Psychiatric Services) Project is described by Peter Barham in his book Closing the Asylum (1992). He reports that, although the discharged patients preferred living in the community and appeared to be developing a more independent view of themselves:

> At one level the pattern of life of the discharged patients did not change very much. In terms of clinical and behavioural measures, for example, there were no significant differences between the leavers and the control group at the end of the year. Similarly, there were few changes in patients' social networks. (p. 22)

There is a current account of the TAPS project in a later chapter of this book.

Another very recent study comparing patients in mental hospital wards with ex-patients in smaller residential facilities 'in the community' reached some similar conclusions. Shepherd and his colleagues from the Sainsbury Centre for Mental Health compared patients in five long-stay psychiatric wards with residents in 20 small community homes for people with mental health problems. The report begins by noting that people with long-term mental health problems have, due to the rundown of mental hospitals, 'experienced profound changes in where they live... with the development of alternative provision in the community'. They propose that the 'Key question is whether they are better off as a result' (Shepherd *et al.*, 1995, p. 5). The answers suggested by the findings are not as unequivocal as the exponents of the literature of dysfunction would have us believe, in that although hospital patients were more disabled, had less pleasant physical environments, lower staffing ratios and more restrictions, nonetheless:

> There was no apparent relationship between levels of dependency and levels of staffing and hospital residents... did not score significantly lower than community residents regarding their feelings of overall well-being or general life satisfaction. (Shepherd *et al.*, 1995, p. 2)

These findings taken together suggest that care in so called 'total institutions' does not inevitably have catastrophic results for its recipients, nor that alternative forms of care in 'community settings' have markedly beneficial results in all respects.

Where there has been comparison in studies such as the Sainsbury Centre one described above, they often do not compare like with like in that they contrast care outcomes for the most disabled patients in old, run-down mental hospitals with outcomes generated for less disabled residents within 'demonstration' projects in the community, which are typically better resourced in all respects. Shepherd *et al.* (1995, p. 1) confirm this suspicion thus:

> Hospital in patients were significantly more impaired on all levels of functioning and dependency [which] supports the idea that a creaming process had taken place, whereby the more able residents had been moved to the community, leaving the more disabled in hospital.

It has yet to be seen whether the frequently only small gains achieved in such projects will be sustained when the researchers go away and the community provision becomes subject to the economic and other resource constraints under which mainstream residential provision has laboured for many years. In this respect, Shepherd and his colleagues come to some interesting conclusions in the final paragraph of their report in relation to the process of 'de-institutionalisation':

> Our findings suggest that we may not have moved as far down the road of understanding this process as we might like to believe... institutional

regimes still exist and staff still continue to behave in institutional ways – even in community settings. These are the really difficult problems that we still have to address. Relocation is just the beginning of the process, it is not an end in itself. (Shepherd *et al.*, 1995, p. 49)

When wider social process is considered in the literature of dysfunction, it often assumes a dualistic form – contrasting the benefits of care in the community with the damaging effects of 'institutionalisation'. Thus in their critique of Townsend's *The Last Refuge*, Jones and Fowles assert that 'The problems of family life were ignored, problems of institutional life were highlighted by contrast' (Jones and Fowles, 1984, p. 85) and that 'The jump from evidence to recommendations is over a sizeable theoretical gap, which Townsend makes no attempt to fill (p. 82). Townsend's criticisms of residential care were contrasted with his vision of reciprocal family care across three generations derived from his study of the family life of old people in the East End of London in the 1950s. The idealistic vision is, of course, now dated (Dobson, 1995, p. 10) and even in its own time frame unrealistic in that the majority of the residents of homes he described had no family. As Jones and Fowles point out, 'By comparison with the elderly in the general population, the institutionalised group had a much higher proportion of the widowed, the divorced and the childless; and that the loss of a close relative usually a husband wife or child often preceded the admission. For a substantial proportion of the sample, three generation reciprocity was not a practical possibility' (p. 85). There is mounting evidence that where old people do live in families, the problems they encounter can include various forms of physical, psychological and financial abuse at least as great as that which has been described in reports on abuse in residential homes (Pritchard, 1992; Eastman, 1994) and evidence too that the effort of caring for severely handicapped elderly relatives can result in family tensions and breakdown. Thus one study of those caring for elderly people with physical disabilities concluded that residential care may be better for both parties than may an increasingly exhausting relationship that can destroy love and affection (Nissel and Bonnerjea, 1982).

Not only is the quality of life of older people unquestioningly assumed to be higher in the community, but also the chances of preserving life itself are alleged to be diminished by leaving it. The so-called 'relocation effect', whereby entry to residential homes is associated with dramatic increases in mortality in elderly people, has added to the rejection of such care by professionals and public alike. However, this 'effect' has been seriously questioned by a series of

American studies employing matched control groups involving almost 1,000 subjects. No evidence was found to support the existence of such a relocation effect, and the authors note that out of the seven previous studies employing matched control groups, six found no corroborative evidence; they concluded:

> There is a need to counter the myth which pervades the nursing home service network that relocation brings about an onslaught of death. (Borup et al., 1979, p. 139)

The tunnel vision and selective neglect of any evidence that casts doubt on the anti-residential care ideology can also be found in relation to child care and mental health. In child care, Bowlby's work on maternal deprivation is often referred to as evidence for the contention that 'a bad family is better than a good institution', despite the fact that later research by Michael Rutter (1981) cast doubt on this belief. His reassessment of Bowlby's work found that substitute parenting – such as that available in children's homes – could provide an adequate emotional experience. More recently, the Wagner Committee, which reviewed residential care for all groups, received evidence that 'some children may prefer residential care to the potential strains and complex demands of foster care' (Sinclair, 1988, p. 45). Despite this, the entrenched view persists that institutional provision is necessarily a poor substitute for family care.

In psychiatry, a similar view of the desirability of family and community care has been fostered by selective reference to the work of 'anti-psychiatrists' such as R.D. Laing, whose powerful critique of psychiatry in the early 1960s proposed that conventional psychiatric treatment oppressively distorted personal experience, re-labelling legitimate protest as insanity in what they described as the 'politics of experience'. However, what they did not do was recommend the abandonment of the asylum; instead they were leading exponents of the therapeutic community movement within which – far from romanticising the superiority of life in family and community – they proclaimed the potential therapeutic value of the asylum as refuge from an insane family, community and indeed society (Laing and Esterson, 1964). Their important writing on the sometimes ruinous effects of family life is similarly conveniently ignored, despite the support lent to it by the later work of Professor Julian Leff and his colleagues from the Institute of Psychiatry, which has described the detrimental effects on schizophrenics of returning to families that demonstrate high levels of expressed emotion (Leff and Vaughn, 1985).

The dualistic conception of 'residential care is bad, community care is good' promoted within the literature of dysfunction neglects these facts. In its narrow focus on the alleged detrimental effects of residential care, it also neglects the fact that the bulk of community care is not provided by formal services created to replace the reviled institutions, but by ordinary people. Thus the value of care provided by informal carers was estimated in 1988 to be between £15 billion and £24 billion, whereas government funds for the implementation of the National Health Service and Community Care Act in 1993 amounted to £539 million (Alzheimer's Disease Society, 1993, pp. 15, 21 and 24). Community care has increasingly been unmasked as care by the family and, within this, care by women. Carers also have rights and choices, which has only recently been recognised in legislation to protect their rights (the Carers [Recognition and Services] Act 1995). This legislation has been prompted by the lobbying of carers' associations – partly as a reaction to the often intolerable burdens imposed on them by the related policies of institutional closure and community care. The anti-institutional lobby has tended to overlook the fact that carers also have rights, and residential provision has been shown to have an important contribution to make to their right to independence and psychological and physical well-being.

A recent report on respite care services for elderly people with dementia from the National Institute for Social Work (Moriarty *et al.*, 1993) found that 'Forty per cent [of the carers] had symptoms of mental distress such as anxiety and depression, associated with high demands and broken nights' and that 'carers looking after the most dependent people were receiving the most intensive services, but these were still quite sparse and inflexible, with little scope for carer choice'. The report concluded that 'Respite services at current levels cannot be presented as an alternative to residential care. For many carers it is only giving up caring which improves their mental health'(National Institute for Social Work, 1993b, pp. 1–2). Another of its findings was that 'Three times as many carers were women than men... almost all the carers felt that caring restricted their lives in some way... nearly all of the caring role fell on the carer alone' (Moriarty *et al.*, 1993, p. 5).

Again, a report from the Alzheimer's Disease Society on carers found a similar concentration of the caring role on women and that community services were often inadequate. Perhaps most ominously in the context of the run down of public residential care, the report found that 35 per cent of carers 'think that they will have to cease caring for their relative at home during the next two to three years'

(Alzheimer's Disease Society, 1993, p. 21). It is within the context of such facts that some feminist writers have also argued for the retention of residential care as a means of promoting the right of women to avoid the oppression of the caring role enforced on them – and internalised by them – through the socially constructed stereotype of femininity (Finch, 1984).

The doubt cast by such studies on the institutionalisation hypothesis and the assumed superiority of care in the community is widely ignored both in the literature of dysfunction and in the 'conventional wisdom' underpinning public policy and professional practice. In a review of several of the most influential works on residential care carried out in the 1980s, Baldwin et al. describe the approach shared by all of them as 'one-dimensional' and overly indebted to the work of early critics such as Goffman and Townsend in that (speaking of one work in particular as exemplary of this) 'They evoke Goffman's concept of the "total institution" as their explanatory framework and view their work as part of a tradition of empirical research which is simply, and straightforwardly, applying Goffman's ideas' (Baldwin et al., 1993, p. 71).

In perhaps the most comprehensive account of the literature of dysfunction, Katherine Jones and A.J. Fowles conclude, in relation to Townsend's work, that it is necessary to 'subtract the detail and the polemic and see what survives in the realm of ideas' (Jones and Fowles, 1984, p. 84) and that 'These hypotheses contained some elements of truth but were both romanticised and sweeping, clichés of sociological thinking rather than rigorous analysis' (p. 83). Ian Sinclair, in an exhaustive review of research into residential care carried out for the Wagner Commission, concluded unequivocally that 'The assertion that past models of care have no value remains unproven' (Sinclair, 1988, p. 52). Unfortunately, despite its many conceptual and methodological shortcomings, the literature of dysfunction has had a considerable influence on the abandonment of public residential provision and the development of the community care movement.

The self-fulfilling prophecy

The anti-residential care movement, in its narrowness of focus, tunnel vision and over-reliance on rhetoric at the expense of scientific rigour, has the characteristics of zealotry and ideology. Rhetoric has proven more persuasive and enduring than reason in promoting the abandonment of this form of care and for the persistence of bias among the helping professions. A recent pronouncement by Professor Michael Oliver could be seen as evidence of this zealotry when he asserted:

> It is worth noting no organisation anywhere in the world which is legitimately entitled to speak for disabled people is advocating residential care for its constituency. Residential care may still have a limited role to play however, because we have to recognise some disabled individuals have been so damaged by what such practice has done to them, that it may be impossible for them to live an independent life. The vast majority of people imprisoned in residential care should be given the support necessary to live in the community... If we are serious about supporting disabled people to live independently, we must acknowledge residential care has no significant role to play in a modern welfare system and is incompatible with the entitlements of citizenship that disabled people are demanding. (Oliver, 1993, p. 13)

Professor Oliver has been an influential critic of residential care and has contributed considerably to thinking about the development of alternative forms of social provision for people with disabilities. Nonetheless, the assertions he makes above lack the sophistication of his wider analysis and cannot be ignored as they are typical of so much of the tunnel vision surrounding the debate. There are, in fact, several organisations for elderly, mentally disabled people and children in Britain who are advocating the retention of residential care as an important element in people's rights as citizens to choice within the care system. See, for example, Age Concern in relation to older people (*Community Care*, 1995, p. 3); The National Society for Mentally Handicapped People in Residential Care (Rescare), which recently published a report on its position (Cox and Pearson, 1995); Schizophrenia a National Emergency (SANE); and the National Schizophrenia Fellowship (NSF). Although now defunct, for many years the National Association of Young People in Care (NAYPIC) was a service user group advocating the retention of residential child care as an essential part of integrated child care provision. Some government bodies too are expressing increasing caution over the continued abandonment of residential provision. The House of Commons Scottish Affairs Committee recently criticised plans to close Scottish mental hospitals, expressing concern about the lack of information on bed numbers, closure policies and alternative provision in the community (Mitchell, 1995). A recent report on residential provision for substance misusers from the Department of Health/Social Services Inspectorate, drawn up after extensive consultation with service providers and user groups, asserted that 'Residential care may be the preferred option most appropriate to meet individual need for one of the following reasons: the service user may need "time out" from an environment which is not conducive to cessation of drug/alcohol misuse; the service user may have a number of complex and inter-related problems which can be addressed only in a residential environment' (Department of Health/Social Services Inspectorate, 1994, p. 7).

Second, as we have seen, much of the evidence for the allegedly harmful effects of residential care is at least questionable.

Finally, Professor Oliver asserts that 'there is no evidence that disabled people freely choose residential care even when they are at their most vulnerable'. It is frequently asserted that because, given the choice, people prefer to live independently in the community, residential care should be abandoned. This is not an argument but a truism. Given the choice, one assumes that people would not choose to enter the operating theatre for surgery; however, this does not lead us to suggest abandoning this form of medical intervention. Given the choice between neglect in the community – which the various reports I have described have shown – and high-quality residential care, I suspect many people would 'choose' the latter.

Having accepted as absolute the questionable assertions of many, albeit eloquent, denunciations of residential care, health and welfare professionals have colluded with a process having all the qualities of the self-fulfilling prophecy. Believing that residential care is an intrinsically undesirable method of intervention, it has come to be used reluctantly as a last resort. As 'treatment' rather than 'tending' is generally the more valued goal of social and medical intervention, there has been a devaluation of the skills involved in providing residential care, which has meant that staff are felt not to require high-level professional training. Despite this, insistence on the superiority of community care has resulted in the conviction that only the most dependent, disturbed or disabled people should enter residential care when all else has failed. As a result, a situation has arisen in which, in the words of one study of residential care for elderly mentally ill people,

> homes have inevitably become surrogate psycho geriatric hospitals without the necessary facilities. (Ovenstone and Bean, 1981, p. 139)

The combination of under-training and inappropriate environments rendered the provision of effective person-oriented care unlikely, and increases in the dependency of clients, beginning in the mid-1970s, placed further pressure on standards of practice in homes. This has sometimes led to those problems associated with low-status work with demanding client groups, carried out in unsuitable buildings – morale has suffered, the task has not been addressed with imagination, care has become routinised and staff and residents have become entrenched, inward-looking and inflexible. The combination of these factors, leading inevitably to poor standards of care, has been termed the 'corruption of care' (Wardhaugh and Wilding, 1993).

An apparently endless series of enquiries into abuse in residential institutions of various types has reinforced the unfavourable assumptions of professionals in health and welfare noted by Barclay (1982) and others. The prophecy has been fulfilled, and this situation has then been attributed to the intrinsic inadequacy of institutional care rather than to the underfunding, poor staff training and inappropriate placement of clients in unsuitable environments. Baldwin *et al.* assert that:

> Conceiving of residential care as a last resort is likely to have reinforced notions of the inevitability of institutionalisation. The social and economic context shaping policies towards residential care, and resources devoted to it, are major predisposing factors in the degree of dependency, independence and interdependence generated. (Baldwin *et al.*, 1993, p. 79)

The anti-residential care bias has indeed been reflected in and reinforced by public policy and legislation throughout the period, such as the 1959 Mental Health Act, the 1963 Children and Young Persons Act, the 1969 Children and Young Persons Act and the 1984 Mental Health Act, all of which stressed the desirability of avoiding institutional care. A series of government reports extolling the virtues of community care for elderly people and other client groups added to the bias, culminating in the National Health Service and Community Care Act 1990, which laid the foundations and provided the financial incentives for the wholesale abandonment of public residential care which has since occurred.

In these ways, publicly provided residential care has been programmed for failure and has now dramatically diminished on the basis of a literature of dysfunction that has limited proof and a social policy of 'community care' that has little established practice. The implications of the debate on residential care have reached far beyond the semantic and theoretical with which we began this chapter. For many thousands of elderly, sick and disabled people, the closure of residential facilities – largely driven by the anti-residential care movement – has led not to care in the community but to abandonment and neglect, not to the extension of choice but to its erosion; and to 'imprisonment' for many not in 'total' institutions but instead in poverty and destitution in the community.

Institutionalisation in the community

The zealotry permeating the anti-residential care movement is further evidenced by its blind assumption of the existence of a 'community'. Sociologists have debated the meaning and nature of community for decades and have reached no consensus on its nature, let alone whether – if it does exist – it is able to or wants to care (Pereira, 1993). Goffman and Barton both stated explicitly that the apparent effects of institutionalisation could be seen in people who had never lived in 'institutions', by which they meant mental hospitals – for example housewives who showed the passivity, apathy and withdrawal that they considered to be symptoms of institutionalisation (Jones and Fowles, 1984, p. 73). This suggestion that institutionalisation was possible in the community has been overlooked by the anti-institution lobby, not only because it undermines their case for closure, but also because their one-dimensional interpretation of the meaning of institution did not enable them to recognise that the family within which housewives exist is also an institution wherein oppressive and depersonalising processes, occur. Feminist writers have consistently exposed these processes, and some, as we have seen, have even advocated residential care as one means by which the oppression of women imprisoned in the socially constructed role of natural carer may be alleviated (Dalley, 1993). Again, caring relatives sometimes display a loss of perspective on the extent of the care that is either possible or needed, and it is not unusual for dedicated carers to enforce an unnecessary dependence on the old person who may then rapidly become de-skilled, losing drive and motivation as a result. This again suggests that some of the alleged aspects of institutionalisation need not necessarily be the result of living in a residential home but can be seen to occur in the community.

More recently, commentators on the failures of community care policy and practice have pointed out how community-based professional practice can lead to institutionalisation in the community. For example, elderly people and those with disabilities living at home may be dependent on domiciliary care services that inadvertently enforce passive conformity to routines designed to serve the organisational exigencies of the providers rather than the individual needs of the recipient (Gavilan, 1992). Thus the National Health Service and Community Care Act 1990 requires social services departments to allocate services according to strict eligibility criteria, which has led to another form of depersonalisation and block treatment. Assessment of need increasingly takes the form of tick lists, usually with a heavy emphasis on functional disability rather than social process, and filled out by the assessor in the role of gatekeeper and 'expert'. Here the number of points allocated by the assessor determines the outcome, rather than there being a holistic, partnership approach involving the service user and affording them some control over the definition of their needs and the nature of the service they require (Smale and Tuson, with Biehal and Marsh, 1993). The 'institution' in this example is the social services bureaucracy and the professional practice associated with it. This is a form of the block treatment said to characterise total institutions and cause institutionalisation and is potentially as depersonalising and oppressive as any experience of residential care.

Other institutions without walls that contribute to the institutionalisation of older people in the community include the institutionalised ageism endemic in Western society (Bytheway, 1995), the structured disadvantage emanating from an economic system that leaves at least 50 per cent of people over 65 in poverty or on the margins of it, and the institution of retirement, which excludes them from sources of income and often brings social exclusion (Townsend, 1993, p. 179). The home lives of frail older people are frequently blighted as much by the poverty and isolation imposed by these institutions as by the physical disabilities they endure, and the personal effects can be identical to those observed in some residential institutions. A study referred to by Baldwin and her colleagues found that 'the proportion of people who sat for hours on end doing nothing in residential care was almost identical to the proportion of people who did so before admission' (Spasoff et al., 1978, in Baldwin et al., 1993, p. 75).The dependency of residents in old people's homes deplored in the literature of dysfunction may well therefore have been socially created long before their admission to residential care, which in the past may have:

> prostitute[d] itself in trying to offer individual cures to problems largely generated by society through poverty, the decaying environment and unemployment. (Walton and Elliott, 1980, p. 22)

Thus, as Baldwin et al. assert:

> Interactive processes may be at work in such situations which may be comparable to those typically regarded as only existing in institutions. (1993, p. 75)

In relation to people with mental illness, Peter Barham, in his book *Closing the Asylum* (1992), similarly points to the way in which professional practice can lead to institutionalisation in the community. He describes the so-called 'aggressive outreach intervention programme' practised as part of the community care of mentally ill people in New

York in which psychiatrists take to the streets and are empowered to remove people compulsorily to emergency rooms for assessment and, if necessary, hospitalisation. Barham asserts that the claims of these practitioners that they are doing something to care for the homeless mentally ill ejected onto the streets by the massive programme of hospital closure belie:

> the essential passivity of this style of intervention: in tearing the culprits off the streets nothing has been done to address the structural deficiencies, not least the need for supported housing, that have at the very least exacerbated the difficulties of former mental patients in the community. (Barham, 1992, p. 48)

Such professional practice is liable to recreate the institutionalised oppression of the mentally ill confined within interactive processes that encourage and enforce dependency, passivity and withdrawal. Referring to the British experience of decarceration, Barham quotes from a study of the views and experiences described by patients discharged from Claybury Hospital in London, the majority of whom saw themselves as being passive recipients of services over which they had no control, one day centre attender saying, 'They're just like being back in hospital, you are not left alone, always being told to do something (Goldie, 1988, in Barham, 1992, p. 61). Another commentator concluded, 'The consequence for consumers has been that most community based provision has replicated the all-too-familiar relationships of institutional life' (Davis, 1988, in Barham, 1992, p. 64).

Barham's analysis is concerned to demonstrate that these problems of replication of paternalistic professional practices and the consequent institutionalisation they bring in the community cannot be resolved by models confined within boundaries of a particular service system. Assumptions underlying the 'institutions are bad, community care is good' dualism hinder the development of new models; Barham asserts that:

> a social process that inclines towards the marginalisation, devaluation and exclusion of mentally disturbed people [and which]... is clearly not a property of the mental hospital but of the operations of a particular kind of society... The elimination of the socially provided option of chronic hospitalisation is hardly likely to resolve the problems vulnerable people encounter in securing a viable social place for themselves. (Barham, 1992, p. 10)

Institutions in community care – a systemic view

In this chapter, I have suggested that the literature of dysfunction is both conceptually limited in its analysis and scientifically flawed in terms of its methodology. There is a gradually mounting critique of this literature and its influence on the development of services for a variety of groups. In relation to psychiatric services, Jones and Fowles (1984) and Jones (1993) provide a detailed analysis, both works exploring this literature and its claims within the history of asylums, their closure and the development of community care policy and practice. In relation to older people and the anti-residential care movement, Baldwin *et al.* (1993) provide a similar critique and come to similar conclusions, as is evident from the title of their paper 'Institutionalisation: why blame the institution?'.

Professor R.A. Parker, in a comprehensive review of the research on residential child care, finds the one-dimensional perspective of the anti-residential care movement similarly limited, its seminal works now so dated as to be virtually irrelevant to current practice and many of its claims ill-supported by much of the more recent research (Parker, 1988a, pp. 3–35; 1988b, pp. 57–124). Cliffe and Berridge, in a study of one local authority in the UK that pursued a radical policy of closing all its children's homes, are cautiously critical of the ideological antipathy towards residential care, which they identified as a major factor in promoting the policy. Having provided a scientifically rigorous analysis of the policy and its practice and given a balanced report of the positive aspects of the policy, the authors nonetheless conclude by urging other authorities to 'think long and hard if they have contemplated repeating what Warwickshire did' (Cliffe and Berridge, 1991, p. 233). All these authors conclude that a more systemic view of the social production of welfare and indeed diswelfare is required if we are to understand the potential role of residential institutions in community care.

Such an approach would have to take into account the interdependence of the various elements of the formal caring services. For example, the closure of long-stay hospital beds for elderly people in the NHS will inevitably have an impact upon residential and nursing homes, at least in terms of the level of demand for places and the needs of the elderly people admitted to them. Failure to acknowledge this will merely lead, as Barham says of similar policies in the psychiatric field, to 'the creation of old problems in new places' (Barham, 1992, p. 143). Ian Sinclair gives an explicit account of the interdependence of these aspects of care provision and asserts that arguments against residential provision generally neglect this. He proposes that residential facilities have numerous advantages: they are robust in that they at least provide minimal care, they have benefits to relatives in assisting them to care, and they have benefits to the welfare system by taking the pressure off domiciliary and other services (Sinclair, 1988, pp. 47–8).

In relation to mental health, Dr Naom Trieman and Professor Julian Leff, in Chapter 2 of this volume, unequivocally conclude that – after a decade of studying the impact of mental hospital closure in London – acute psychiatric services are being overwhelmed by the unforeseen and unplanned-for consequences of de-institutionalisation, with 100 per cent plus occupancy of acute facilities. They conclude that the 'difficult-to-place' and the 'new long-stay' psychiatric patients will always be with us and will always require some form of asylum in long-term care facilities.

In the child care field, Professor Parker gives a detailed analysis of the balance of care between fostering and residential provision and argues convincingly that it will neither be possible nor desirable to close children's homes. This is because the maintenance of the system of foster care is reliant on a certain level of residential provision being available, even if only to provide short-term care for the one in five foster placements that he estimates breaks down annually. He proposes that, in order to maintain the level of foster care placement current in 1984 (38,000 children), 2,850 children's home places will be required each year. Parker asserts that 'Whether or not the figures and assumptions in this illustrative example are exactly right they serve to draw attention to the relationship between foster care and residential care in a way that is relevant to planning' (Parker, 1988b, pp. 70–1). Whilst this interdependence seems self-evident, it has largely been ignored in the flight from public residential provision for all client groups.

The systemic model must then extend beyond the boundaries of individual services and their relationship to the wider community and the institutions of all types that provide care within it. It must take into account both those services formally designated as 'caring' and others such as housing, leisure, transport, libraries and education, all of which are involved in the social production of welfare and diswelfare, all of which may promote either dependence or independence in individuals and all of which are in fact interdependent as institutions. Thus, for example, the logic and viability of a policy of closing public residential provision for older people at a time when the institution of the family is least able to provide care is questionable.

As is well documented, economic and demographic factors such as mass unemployment, fewer single women, more female participation in the paid workforce and higher levels of divorce all undermine the ability of the family to provide care and add to the burden of those who manage to do so. To neglect this in the formulation of policy and the implementation of practice will inevitably lead to the premature collapse of informal care provision in the family, as a recent study by the Alzheimer's Disease Society found, with one in five carers saying that they would definitely not be able to continue caring. One of the reasons for this was the widespread financial and material deprivation among elderly people and their carers, in part due to a benefits system that:

> makes it almost impossible for carers to combine caring with part-time work [and] discriminates against older people many of whom have given up work early in order to care. (Alzheimer's Disease Society, 1993, p. 20).

One carer interviewed in the study estimated that, as a direct result of recent government policies on elderly families with mentally impaired dependants, the extra costs of caring have increased by £2,585 per annum. This is further evidence of a failure to take a systemic view of the social production of welfare in the community, in that the role of the institutions of compulsory retirement and social security in promoting dependence has been neglected. Similar analyses have been applied to the interdependence of housing policy and housing benefits in relation to the success or failure of community care (Yanetta and Naumann, 1994; Griffiths, 1995). The massive loss of publicly provided residential care is likely further to undermine the ability of the family to care, as there is evidence that the availability of residential respite care is central to the continuation of family care in the community. Private providers are less likely to offer such services in view of the under-occupancy of beds and the consequent loss of income that is entailed. The survey conducted by the National Institute for Social Work referred to earlier concluded that:

> Carers who had been using [residential] relief care for some time were extremely unlikely to have opted for [permanent] residential care in the near future. (1993b, p. 3)

These facts suggest that government policy in the UK is, in some ways, promoting the production of diswelfare in the community rather than promoting the ability of the community to care. Central to this has been the dualistic conception of the role of residential institutions in community care that has prevailed among professionals and policy makers for the past 30 years, and the abandonment of publicly provided residential and hospital care for elderly, sick and disabled people which it has promoted. Zealotry and ideology are inadequate substitutes for reasoned analysis; nonetheless, the consequences of this ill-supported moral outrage have been borne by hundreds of thousands of mentally ill, old and disabled people over the past 30 years. Peter Barham describes it thus:

> As we have seen here these various forms of loss [of identity, status and opportunity] may occur just as easily outside the asylum as within it... community care has among other things provided new opportunities for betrayal in the relationship between service providers and people with mental illness. (Barham, 1992, p. 60)

The revisionist backlash in residential care

This betrayal is not limited to the replication in the community of the oppressive and depersonalising practice of the worst form of residential provision described by Barham, Jones, Baldwin and others. An equally damaging betrayal is the abandonment of the discipline and professional practice of residential care to colonisation by the piratical and punitive. There is now gathering momentum a revisionist backlash – a re-institutionalisation movement dominated by extreme right-wing politicians and commercial interests intent on either reducing taxation of the rich by cutting public expenditure or promoting their own personal wealth through the commoditisation of the elderly and mentally ill, aided by government policies designed to develop a 'mixed economy of welfare'. The policy of closure of publicly provided old people's homes in Britain, and a social security payments system that funded private care for older and disabled people, has led to a massive growth in the private residential care sector of 130 per cent between 1979 and 1990 such that most such provision is now within the independent sector. Residential care for older people has become big business, and, as commodities within it, old people have fallen victim to market forces, with numerous accounts of the eviction of old people from such facilities when their ability to fund this care is exhausted (Whiteley, 1995, pp. 8 and 9). Professor Bleddyn Davies – who has been a leading proponent of community care policy formulation in the UK over the past two decades – has warned against the possible 'pauperisation' of a generation of older people within this system (Davies, 1990). The availability of a publicly provided welfare safety net for these victims of market forces is continually being eroded through the underfunding of care in the community – the Association of County Councils estimating that the shortfall would amount to £400 million in 1995 (Downey, 1994, p. 1) – and social services departments charged with implementing it are said to be in crisis and 'disillusioned with the community care policy' (Marchant, 1995, p. 16).

In relation to recarceration in mental health, the American experience has been that the social problems of the thousands of chronic mental patients precipitately discharged from state mental hospitals closed under the de-institutionalisation programme have led to a backlash in public opinion characterised by intolerance and fear, and measures, aimed at reassuring the public, that are little short of punitive. In major cities, thousands of homeless and disordered individuals are being housed in 'shelters' with minimal facilities and are policed by psychiatric professionals whose main function seems to be to reassure the public that such people will be rapidly removed from the streets and 'assertively' treated in overcrowded short-term care facilities that often replicate the worst features of the old state mental hospitals (Barham, 1992, p. 120). What is referred to as the 'jail explosion' in the USA has been partly fuelled by increasingly punitive attitudes towards mentally disordered offenders, increasing numbers of whom find themselves incarcerated in prison rather than a mental hospital. A graphic description of the re-institutionalisation movement in California – once in the vanguard of decarceration and community care – is given by Wolch et al. (1988), who discuss the 'unfulfilled promise of de-institutionalisation', the mass homelessness and poverty of ex-patients, the public fear and intolerance of this and the consequent pressures for 'increasing social control' through community treatment orders and recarceration, either in prisons or reopened and often inadequate 'shelters'. They unequivocally assert that:

> The concept of deinstitutionallisation was flawed by the notion that serious, chronic mental disorders could be minimised... through care provided within the local community. The community care paradigm was never sufficiently validated, despite its emergence as the conceptual and ideological basis for mental health policy. (Wolch et al., 1988, p. 35)

The authors describe how the movement 'back to the backwards' is well underway in California.

Similar disastrous consequences of the decarceration movement in Italy are reviewed by Professor Jones in her book *Asylums and After* (1993). Law no. 180, passed after intense political pressure by left-wing movements in 1978, abolished mental hospitals and proposed the establishment of alternative community treatment centres. However, two study tours undertaken by Jones in the late 1980s disclosed the massive failure of this programme, with homelessness of ex-patients (known in Italy as the *abbandonati*), inadequate community resources, and virtually unrecognised and poorly funded residual back wards in the old hospitals still in use. She found that:

> Psychiatrists, psychiatric nurses and social workers described how Law no. 180 had created an avalanche of apparently insuperable problems. (Jones, 1993, p. 220).

Jones poses the question of why 'politically biased accounts of the Italian experience, based on very selective information', have been so influential in promoting the decarceration movement in Britain and concludes that an unholy and inadvertent alliance of well-intentioned reformers and right-wing politicians intent on reducing public expenditure offers some explanation. She concludes that:

> In the event, the only lessons for Britain are that extreme left wing reform movements can very easily be turned to right wing ends, and that it is much easier to destroy the existing services than to create better ones. (Jones, 1993, p. 221).

As I have attempted to show in this chapter, the selective use of biased information has characterised the anti-residential care movement in the UK, and similar dire consequences have emerged, as the letter from Prime Minister John Major referred to in my introduction to this book shows. His assertion that the closure programme 'may have gone too far' is a belated recognition of the consequences of the flight from public residential provision for people with mental health problems – one which will be of little help to the thousands of seriously disordered patients ejected into poverty and destitution in communities that are either not able or not willing to care through a community care policy, fuelled by what Jones has termed the 'ideologies of destruction'.

Both welfare and diswelfare are socially produced. Similar systemic processes dominated by professional aspiration and political ideology produced the reviled workhouse, children's homes, asylums and the revered policies of decarceration and 'community care'. The 'institutions' involved in the production of welfare are many and varied, as I have suggested; they all have the potential for the personal growth or depersonalisation of the individuals within them. The adverse effects of 'institutionalisation' can occur in residential care and in the community. Today, dualistic concepts of this production of welfare, which damn one institution and deify another, are unhelpful and limiting. The sooner we develop realistic models of how communities care that are capable of addressing this and other facets of the social production of welfare, the sooner the well-documented misery of these mentally ill, disabled and older citizens of our societies will be alleviated.

References

Alzheimer's Disease Society (1993) *Deprivation and Dementia*. London, Alzheimer's Disease Society.

Audit Commission (1985) *Managing Social Services for the Elderly More Effectively*. London, HMSO.

Baldwin, N., Harris, J. and Kelly, D. (1993) Institutionalisation: why blame the institution? *Ageing and Society*, **13**:69–81.

Barclay, P. (1982) *Social Workers: Their Role and Tasks. Report of a Working Party*. London, Bedford Square Press.

Barham, P. (1992) *Closing the Asylum*. London, Penguin.

Barton, R. (1959) *Institutional Neurosis*. Bristol, John Wright.

Booth, T. (1985) *Home Truths. Old People's Homes and the Outcome of Care*. Aldershot, Gower.

Bornat, J., Pereira, C., Pilgrim, D. and Williams, F. (eds) (1993) *Community Care: A Reader*. Basingstoke, Macmillan and Buckingham, Open University Press.

Borup, J.H., Gallego, D.T. and Heffernan, P.G. (1979) Relocation and its effects on mortality. *Gerontologist*. **19**(2):135–40.

Bowlby, J. (1969) *Attachment and Loss*, vol. 1. *Attachment*. London, Hogarth Press.

Bytheway, B. (1995) *Ageism*. Buckingham, Open University Press.

Cliffe, D. and Berridge, D. (1991) *Closing Children's Homes: An End to Residential Care?* London, National Childrens Bureau.

Clough, R. (1981) *Old Age Homes*. London, Allen & Unwin.

Community Care (1995) Too many elderly people live in care. 26 January:3.

Cox, C. and Pearson, M. (1995) *Made to Care. The Case for Residential and Village Communities for People with Mental Handicap*. London, Rannoch Trust.

Dalley, G. (1993) The principles of collective care, in Bornat, J. *et al.*, *op. cit.*, pp. 152–5.

Davies, B. (1990) The trade and industry metaphor and its relevance to the Griffiths Report, in Bytheway, B. and Johnson, J. (eds) *The Ageing Experience*. Aldershot, Gower, pp. 14–27.

Davis, A. (1988) Users' perspectives, in Ramon, S. with Giannicheda, M. (eds) *Psychiatry in Transition*. London, Pluto Press, quoted in Barham, P. *op. cit.*

Department of Health (1981) *Report on a Study on Community Care*. London, HMSO.

Department of Health/Social Services Inspectorate (1994) *Residential Care for People with Drug/Alcohol Problems: A Report of a Consultative Project*. London, HMSO.

Dobson, R. (1995) Only the lonely. *Community Care*, 29 June–5 July:10.

Downey, R. (1994) Budget revives fears of cash cuts. *Community Care*, 1–7 December:1.

Eastman, M. (ed.) (1994) *Old Age Abuse: A New Perspective*. London, Chapman & Hall.

Elkan, R. and Kelly, D. (1991) *A Window in Homes: Links Between Residential Care Homes and the Community – A Literature Review*. Surbiton, Residential Care Association.

Falkingham, J. (1989) Dependency and ageing in Britain: a re-examination of the evidence. *Journal of Social Policy*, **18**(2): 211–33.

Finch, J. (1984) Community care: developing non-sexist alternatives. *Critical Social Policy*, **9**:6–18.

Flemming, J. and Oppenheimer, P. (1996) Are Government spending and taxes too high (or too low)? *National Institute Economic Review*, **31**(7).

Gavilan, H. (1992) Taking control from the frail. *Guardian*, 17 June.

Goffman, E. (1961) *Asylums: Essays on the Social Situation of Mental Patients and Other Inmates*. New York, Anchor Books/Doubleday.

Goldie, N. (1988) I hated it there but I miss the people: a study of what has happened to a group of ex-long stay patients from Claybury Hospital. London, South Bank Polytechnic Health and Social Services Research Unit, research paper no. 1., quoted in Barham, P. *op. cit.*

Griffiths, Sir R. (1988) *Community Care: Agenda for Action* (The Griffiths Report). London, HMSO.

Griffiths, S. (1995) Discouraging independence. *Community Care*, 29 June–5 July:26–7.

Henderson, P. and Armstrong, J. (1993) Community development and community care: a strategic approach, in Bornat, J. *et al. op. cit.*, pp. 327–34.

Hills, J. (ed.) (1990) *The State of Welfare*. Oxford, Oxford University Press.

Johnstone, E.C., Owens, D.G.C., Gold, A. *et al.* (1981) Institutionalisation and the defects of schizophrenia. *British Journal of Psychiatry*, **139**:195–203.

Jones, K. (1993) *Asylums and After. A Revised History of the Mental Health Services: From the Early 18th Century to the 1990s*. London, Athlone Press.

Jones, K. and Fowles, A.J. (1984) *Ideas on Institutions. Analysing the Literature on Long Term Care and Custody*. London, Routledge & Kegan Paul.

Laing, R.D. and Esterson, A. (1964) *Sanity, Madness and the Family*. London, Tavistock.

Leff, J.P. and Vaughn, C.E. (1985) *Expressed Emotion in Families: Its Significance for Mental Illness*. London, Guildford Press.

McCarthy, M. (1989) *The New Politics of Welfare*. Basingstoke, Macmillan.

Marchant, C. (1995) Hard times. *Community Care*, 26 January–1 February:16.

Meacher, M. (1972) *Taken for a Ride*. London, Longman.

Miller, E.J. and Gwynne, G.V. (1972) *A Life Apart. A Pilot Study of Residential Institutions for the Physically Handicapped and young Chronic Sick*. London, Tavistock.

Mitchell, D. (1995) Psychiatric hospitals plan slammed by MPs. *Community Care*, 29 June–5 July:2.

Moriarty, J., Levin, E. and Gorbach, I. (1993) *Respite Services for Carers of Confused Elderly People*. London, National Institute for Social Work.

Morris, P. (1969) *Put Away: A Sociological Study of Institutions for the Mentally Retarded*. London, Routledge & Kegan Paul.

National Institute for Social Work (1993a) *Positive Answers*. London, HMSO.

National Institute for Social Work (1993b) Policy Briefings No.1, October.

Nissel, M. and Bonnerjea, L. (1982) *Family Care of the Handicapped Elderly: Who Pays?* London, Policy Studies Institute.

Oliver, M. (1993) Struggling for independence. *Community Care*, 2 September:13.

Ovenstone, I.R.K. and Bean, P. (1981) A medical, social assessment of admissions to old peoples' homes in Nottingham. *British Journal of Psychiatry*, **139**:226–9.

Parker, R.A. (1988a) An historical background to residential care, in Sinclair I., *op. cit.*, pp. 3–38.

Parker, R.A. (1988b) Residential care for children, in Sinclair, I. *op. cit.*, pp. 57–124.

Pereira, C. (1993) Anthology: the breadth of community, in Bornat, J. *et al.*, *op. cit.*, pp. 5–20.

Pritchard, J. (1992) *The Abuse of Elderly People: A Handbook for Professionals*. London, Jessica Kingsley.

Robb, B. (1967) *Sans Everything: A Case to Answer*. London, Nelson.

Rutter, M. (1981) *Maternal Deprivation Reassessed*. Harmondsworth, Penguin.

Seebohm, Sir F. (1968) *Report of the Committee on Local Authority and Allied Personal Social Services* (The Seebohm Report). London, HMSO.

Shepherd, G., Muijen, M., Dean, R. *et al.* (1995) *Inside Residential Care: The Realities of Hospital Versus Community Settings*. London, Sainsbury Centre for Mental Health.

Sinclair, I. (ed.) (1988) *Residential Care: the Research Reviewed*. London, HMSO.

Smale, G. and Tuson, G., with Biehal, N. and Marsh, P. (1993) *Empowerment, Assessment, Care Management and the Skilled Worker*. London, HMSO.

Spasoff, R.A., Kraus, A.S, Beattie, E.J. *et al.* (1978) A longitudinal study of elderly residents of long stay institutions. *Gerontologist*, **18**:281–92.

Tobin, S. and Lieberman, M.A. (1976) *Last Home for the Aged*. San Francisco, Jossey Bass.

Townsend, P. (1962) *The Last Refuge*. London, Routledge & Kegan Paul.

Townsend, P. (1993) The structured dependency of the elderly: a creation of social policy in the 20th century, in Bornat, J. *et al.*, *op. cit.*, pp. 178–83.

Wagner, G. (1988) *Residential Care: A Positive Choice* (The Wagner Report). London, National Institute for Social Work.

Walton, R.G. and Elliott, D. (eds) (1980) *Residential Care: A Reader in Current Theory and Practice*. Oxford, Pergamon Press.

Wardhaugh, J. and Wilding, P. (1993) Towards an explanation of the corruption of care. *Critical Social Policy*, **13**(37): ?.

Webster, P. (1996) Age time bomb is alarmist myth, MPs tell ministers. *Times*, 8 August:2.

Whiteley, P. (1995) Residents booted out as care gap grows. *Community Care*, 3 March–5 April:8, 9.

Willcocks, D., Peace, S. and Kellaher, L. (1987) *Private Lives in Public Places*. London, Tavistock.

Wistow, G. and Barnes, M. (1993) User involvement in community care: user involvement and applications. *Public Administration*, Autumn: 71.

Wolch, J.R., Nelson, C.A. and Rubalcabaca, A. (1988) Reinstitutionalisation of the mentally disabled, in Smith, C.J. and Giggs, J.A. (eds) *Location and Stigma. Contemporary Perspectives on Mental Health and Mental Health Care.* Boston, Unwin Hyman, p. 35.

Yanetta, A. and Naumann, L. (1994) No housing – no community care, in Davidson, R. and Hunter, S. (eds) *Community Care in Practice.* London, Batsford, pp. 55–63.

2 CLOSING PSYCHIATRIC HOSPITALS – SOME LESSONS FROM THE TAPS PROJECT

Naom Trieman and Julian Leff

The previous chapter described and discussed the critique of residential care and, drawing on recent research findings from the UK, USA and Italy in relation to the closure of residential institutions for people with mental illness, old people and other groups, pointed to both the inadequacy of the critique and the results of the policy and practice based upon it. It offered a systemic view of the place of residential institutions in caring communities. This chapter describes one of the most comprehensive longitudinal studies of psychiatric hospital closure in the UK. It has been concerned to pursue a systemic view of community care and has found that much is gained in terms of meeting the needs of people with mental health problems by providing community-based services. However, it has also established that intense pressure is placed by such policies on other elements of the care system in communities, and that, if the needs of people with mental health problems are to be met and if the system as a whole is to function adequately, long-term residential facilities for thousands of people with severe mental disorder will always be required.

The TAPS project: an introduction

In 1983 North East Thames Regional Health Authority (NETRHA) announced a 10 year programme to close two of its six psychiatric hospitals, Friern and Claybury. The policy to be pursued was innovative at that time, because there was no intention of decanting patients into other psychiatric hospitals, as had been done before with the closure of similar hospitals. Instead the aim was to reprovide all hospital services within the community.

This was seen as a unique opportunity to mount a comprehensive evaluation of the policy and its implementation. The Team for the Assessment of Psychiatric Services (TAPS) was established in 1985 with funding contributions from NETRHA, the King's Fund and the Department of Health. TAPS set itself a broad agenda of research (O'Driscoll and Leff, 1993). The main objective was to evaluate the clinical and social outcomes of long-stay patients discharged into the community. A short-term (1 year) follow-up study was recently concluded, while a long-term (5 years) outcome study is still ongoing.

Other aspects associated with the reprovision programme were evaluated as well. The processes of decision making in statutory agencies, a crucial factor affecting the success of reprovision, were monitored throughout the programme (Thomlinson, 1991). The effects of the changes on relatives, staff and the community were evaluated in a series of studies (Dayson, 1993; Reda, 1993). The impact produced by the closure of Friern Hospital on the district acute admission services was formally monitored (Sammut, 1992). An economic analysis was integrated with the clinical studies to assess the cost implications of the closure programme. This has been carried out by a team of health economists from the Personal and Social Services Research Unit (PSSRU) (Knapp et al., 1993).

Notions on the main results

The TAPS study has clearly shown that the majority of the long-stay patients discharged from psychiatric hospitals benefited from moving to the community (Leff et al., 1996). Most patients, with the exception of a small group of people called 'difficult to place', have settled successfully within a range of supported accommodation (Lewis and Trieman, 1995; Trieman and Kendal, 1995). The houses, most of which are staffed group homes, provide a domestic environment in which residents have their own bedroom and can enjoy freedom from the many inherent restrictions imposed on them in hospital. These changes were greatly appreciated by the patients (Leff et al., 1996). Some of the patients gained more friends in the community, yet social interactions between patients and members of the public generally remain few and far between.

Overall, the mental state, social behaviour and basic living skills of the former long-stay patients have shown little change over the first year of follow-up (Leff *et al.*, 1996). At the 5 year follow-up, these outcomes seem to be sustainable (Leff *et al.*, 1994). Rates of crime, vagrancy and mortality – major areas of concern for the public and care providers – were reassuringly low (Dayson, 1993).

The least satisfactory part of the Friern reprovision programme was the planning of the alternative admission facilities. The closure programme was used seemingly as an opportunity to reduce the total number of admission beds within the catchment area (Sammut, 1992). Following the closure of Friern Hospital, the occupancy of admission beds in two of the health districts regularly exceeded 100 per cent.

This crisis situation is not unique to the area of North London. Indeed, there is substantial evidence that the practice of providing insufficient numbers of acute beds is becoming a nationwide problem (Powell and Hollander, 1994). The scarcity of medium-term rehabilitation facilities disadvantages those patients who are less responsive to treatment (Bridges *et al.*, 1994), many of whom are currently 'blocking' acute wards throughout the country (Lelliot and Wing, 1994, I, II).

The TAPS study pointed at one contributary factor to the bed crisis, which is a direct consequence of reprovision, namely the ongoing need of resettled patients for readmission. On average, 15 per cent of the patients discharged following the closure of Friern hospital were readmitted at least once during the first year of follow-up (Gooch and Leff, 1996). It was estimated that, at any one time, nine beds were needed per 100 discharged long-stay patients to cater for their admission needs. Whilst this crude estimate can hardly be generalized, it indicates a factor that should not be overlooked in the planning of admission services within a catchment area.

Another aspect about which we have learnt from the experience of closing psychiatric hospitals in England is that, regardless of locality, structure or quality of community psychiatric services, a small proportion of the long-term hospital population will always need some sort of continuous inpatient care. Evidently, any reprovision programme for a psychiatric hospital is bound to face a serious challenge of how to reprovide for a residual group of severely disabled patients for whom adequate care within the community is impossible. TAPS has launched a series of research projects to study the characteristics and outcomes of these difficult-to-place patients (Dayson *et al.*, 1992; Trieman and Leff, 1996, a, b). The findings are presented below.

The 'difficult to place'

Throughout the course of the reprovision programme for Friern Hospital, a group of long-stay patients, previously discharged from Friern Hospital, along with a number of newly admitted patients, have accumulated in hospital and remained for longer than a year (Dayson, 1993). A proportion of this 'new long-stay' population, together with a group of residual 'old long-stay' patients (some of whom had spent virtually all their lives in hospital), constituted the core group of patients who were considered too difficult to place in the community.

Seventy-two Friern patients, designated by the hospital staff as 'difficult to place', were transferred shortly before the hospital closed to four specialised care facilities (instead of ordinary community homes). This group constituted 14 per cent of the hospital long-stay population (as it was in 1985). The figure implies a prevalence of 10–11 difficult-to-place patients per 100,000 of the general population in the region of north London.

Each of the patients identified as 'difficult to place' underwent a comprehensive psychiatric and social assessment shortly before leaving hospital. The group of difficult-to-place patients were then compared with the rest of the long-stay population, which consisted of patients who settled successfully over the years within the available range of community facilities.

Characteristics of the 'difficult to place'

The baseline study (Trieman and Leff, 1996a) showed that patients identified as 'difficult to place' were relatively young, the majority male, with a shorter duration of stay in comparison with the rest of the hospital population. Although not excessively disabled functionally or physically, the difficult-to-place patients were slightly more disturbed in their mental state. The more distinctive features of the 'difficult to place' were associated with disruptive modes of behaviour. A cluster of serious behavioural problems were designated by staff as a direct impediment in placing a patient in a community home. The most common problem areas were aggressiveness (both verbal and physical), non-compliance with treatment and inappropriate sexual behaviour.

Clusters of challenging behaviours similar to the one identified by TAPS have been given in the past by other studies (Gudeman and Shore, 1984; Bigelow *et al.*, 1988; Cane Hill Research Team, 1991). Focusing on problematic behaviours, rather than aspects such as poor functioning, is based on the realisation that, whilst the most withdrawn patients are still manageable in highly supported homes, certain aspects of behaviour, notably physical aggression, are perceived as intolerable in this context. Whilst challenging problems are clearly non-specific, they are over-represented and reach extreme levels among the difficult-to-place patients, hence making them hard to control in a hospital and even harder to manage, if at all possible, within a less structured environment (for example a group home).

The 'new long-stay'

Patients with severe persisting illnesses, who are difficult to manage within the community, are not going to vanish along with the psychiatric hospitals. In fact, all the evidence shows that patients continue to accumulate in psychiatric wards, either in existing psychiatric hospitals or in district general hospitals. This phenomenon was observed during the early stages of running down hospitals in the UK (Mann and Cree, 1976; Wykes and Wing, 1982), and it soon became apparent in the course of the TAPS follow-up study (Thornicroft *et al.*, 1992). Notably, two-thirds of the difficult-to-place group at Friern Hospital consisted of patients who by definition were 'new long-stay'.

Socially deprived catchment areas, particularly inner cities, are associated with higher accumulation rates and consequently with a higher prevalence of 'new long-stay' patients (Thornicroft *et al.*, 1992; Lelliot and Wing, 1994, I, II). In certain places, the insufficiency of alternative facilities in the community simply means that more newly admitted patients are retained in hospital. However, even with the best existing range of community care provisions, it is all too clear that, if long-term inpatient care is unavailable, these so-called 'new long-stay' patients will be the most likely people to drift into homelessness or be criminalised. The acceleration of the 'revolving door' phenomenon, along with the revelation that one-third of the acute beds in the UK are occupied by 'new long-stay' patients (Lelliot and Wing, 1994, I, II) is indeed a worrying sign.

Provisions for the 'difficult to place'

In the UK, where the local health authorities are committed to providing a comprehensive range of community services to replace the psychiatric hospital, a pressing dilemma has arisen for the planners in deciding which types of setting would optimally meet the heterogeneous needs of patients identified as 'difficult to place'. Should the solution be in the form of a specialised, domestic-type rehabilitation unit? This type of setting, although providing a better quality of life, is quite expensive and might not suit the needs of all difficult-to-place patients, thus compelling the purchasers to buy hospital services from providers elsewhere. Alternatively, should the solution be a replication of the traditional continuing care ward? This is certainly a less expensive solution with no pretence of active rehabilitation but one still capable of containing most of the difficult-to-place patients.

The dilemma is complex, involving economic, therapeutic and moral considerations (hopefully not in that order). Furthermore, in planning alternative facilities for the residual group of difficult-to-place patients, one must also envisage the future needs of a new generation of chronic patients in an era when psychiatric hospitals may no longer exist. These needs would not necessarily be the same as for those currently designated 'difficult to place'.

If we put aside the economic considerations and first explore what optimal therapeutic environment might suit difficult-to-place patients, we find that there is a substantial amount of evidence to indicate that hostel wards provide an effective form of care for highly disabled patients (Garety and Morris, 1984; Gibbons, 1986; Hyde *et al.*, 1987; Allen *et al.*, 1993; Shepherd *et al.*, 1994; Shepherd, 1995). The model of a 'ward in a house', originally formulated by Douglas Bennet (1980), was designed to combine the best features of hospital care (good staffing levels and well-trained professionals) with the best features of community-based residential care (small, domestic in nature and accessible to the community) (Wykes and Wing, 1982; Goldberg *et al.*, 1985; Shepherd *et al.*, 1994). Curiously, as pointed out by Shepherd (1995), this model is reminiscent of one of the very first institutions for the mentally ill, the York Retreat, founded in 1796. Progressive it might well be, yet the 'ward in a house' model is certainly less innovative than one might be led to believe.

The target population for a 'ward in a house' type setting is primarily the 'new long-stay' patients (Wykes and Wing, 1982; Young, 1991). In this respect, such a facility seems to be of particular relevance to the needs of people designated as 'difficult to place'.

However, some questions are bound to arise: Can a hostel ward meet the heterogeneous needs of the difficult-to-place patients? Is it capable of promoting the functional skills of these patients? Can it modify the patients' challenging modes of behaviour? Is it a cost-effective option?

Currently, the number of beds in hostel wards within the UK is 3.7 per 100,000 members of the population – less than 6 per cent of the total inpatient beds (Lelliot and Wing, 1994). There are quite a few variations among these settings with regard to the administration, principles of care and target populations, thus making comparison of outcomes a somewhat problematic task. In general, however, most of these settings are hospital based, providing medium-term accommodation and employing a basic rehabilitation programme. Shepherd (1995), who summarised outcome data from 'ward in a house' facilities, reached the conclusion that these units were more effective in improving social functioning and maintaining activity levels than were traditional psychiatric hospital wards.

Whilst there is some evidence that most of these facilities are indeed successful in engaging their patients in constructive activity and in utilising community amenities, reports are less consistent with regard to social functioning and the performance of living skills. An evaluative study of Douglas House in Manchester, one of the country's best-known hostel wards (Goldberg et al., 1985; Hyde et al., 1987), shows that the residents did not improve their social and self-care performance, yet they gained better domestic skills.

The TAPS study (Trieman and Leff, 1996b) evaluated the outcomes of difficult-to-place patients in three types of hostel ward. We found that, regardless of the different milieu and rehabilitation input, there had not been any overall significant change in the level of social or self-care functioning. We therefore believe that one should not expect substantial gains in this field. A key issue is whether specialised units for the 'difficult to place' have the potential to modify some of the most disruptive behaviours that impede the patients' progress. This aspect of care effectiveness is bound to determine the patients' future more than anything else.

The TAPS study demonstrates (Trieman and Leff, 1996b) that the profile of serious behaviour problems amongst difficult-to-place patients is not static. Aggressive behaviour – undoubtedly the most serious problem – proved to be potentially reversible. This was particularly apparent in one of the facilities, a fine example of a 'ward in a house', employing non-restrictive and flexible non-intrusive attitudes. It succeeded in lessening the overall frequency of problem behaviours and most notably managed to reduce the levels of aggression (both verbal and physical). These findings should serve as an incentive for care planners to explore ways of modifying challenging behaviours, instead of directing all the rehabilitation efforts to the acquisition of living skills, which seem to be unrewarding with regard to difficult-to-place patients.

Whilst we generally regard the hostel ward as probably the best environment for the majority of patients with challenging behaviours, it is not, however, the optimal environment for all difficult-to-place patients. Some of them might react adversely to growing levels of freedom and increasing expectations, and thus might fare better with stricter boundaries. A sizable minority are too difficult to manage within a domestic environment and are excessively disruptive in the neighbourhood. These individuals usually exhibit the highest levels of aggression and extreme acting-out behaviour, which can pose a degree of danger. Most reports show that up to one-third of patients referred to hostel wards are eventually transferred to a more secure setting (Shepherd, 1995). Based on the TAPS evaluation, specialised facilities have a greater potential to succeed in containing some of the most difficult patients. Notably, the least restrictive facility of the four units studied by TAPS has managed to contain all but two of its 28 residents, of whom half were consistently aggressive.

The variety of care environments needed for difficult-to-place patients was discussed by Gudeman and Shore (1984), who suggested that a cluster of specialised units should be located in the grounds of a large campus and provide for the entire difficult-to-place population within a region or even a whole state. We do not favour this option, since it practically means a revival of the old institutional model. Instead we recommend that every reprovision programme should set up one or more hostel wards in the locality, depending on the prevalence of difficult-to-place patients (Trieman and Leff, 1996a). From a managerial point of view, it seems more practical to situate such units in the grounds of a general hospital or next to an existing psychiatric hospital. It is perfectly viable, however, to place special care units in the community, provided they maintain close links with a nearby hospital. In order to accommodate the heterogeneous needs, it is advisable to establish two to three specialised units (or divide one unit into subunits), which will differ in the degree of structuring, social contact and rehabilitative endeavour. The units should be intensively staffed, as we regard this as a precondition for the feasibility of an 'open door' policy and for the delivery of good practice.

Economic considerations

Providing services for the difficult-to-place patients is expensive, as shown by the economic study conducted in parallel with the main TAPS study (Hallam, 1996). The economic evaluation of the Friern reprovision programme shows that the weekly care package for a person identified as 'difficult to place' was, on average, £1,065 (at 1994–95 price levels). An expensive capital programme had been undertaken in two of the settings that were planned for the difficult-to-place group, and high numbers of qualified staff were employed. Twenty-four hour waking cover was provided by each of the three units. Ninety-four per cent of the total cost is accounted for by services provided within the accommodation facility.

In comparison, the mean cost of care for former long-stay Friern Hospital patients (not including this group) was £612 per week. It must be remembered that many of the earlier leavers were able to move to independent accommodation, or to units with lower staffing levels, whilst the residual hospital patients were more dependent. The difference between the later amount and the average costs for those identified as 'difficult to place' reflects the particular challenges presented by patients with severe problems.

With only a few exceptions (e.g. Allen, 1993), specialised facilities for difficult-to-place patients are intensively staffed and thus very expensive (Hallam, 1991). The cost of a hospital–hostel type of setting is estimated to be the same as that of an acute ward in a district general hospital and nearly double the cost of the so-called 'back' wards in mental hospitals (Young, 1991). It is obvious that the total cost of reprovision for the whole hospital population is significantly affected by the expensive provisions needed for the difficult-to-place group. In fact, it is estimated that the cost contribution of providing for the difficult to place has made 'care in the community' an overall more dear option than care within the hospital (Hallam, 1996). The next inevitable question is therefore: are these facilities cost-effective?

Two of the settings assessed by TAPS (Trieman and Leff, 1996a) were highly resourced, with a nursing staff:patient ratio as high as 1.7:1. Comparison with less well-resourced facilities, based on parameters of containment and rehabilitation, reveals that costly facilities for difficult-to-place patients are no guarantee of better outcomes. Why, then, should we invest in expensive settings and not opt for cheaper options? This is a matter of judgement rather than solely a scrutiny of cost-effectiveness. We believe that the absence of restrictive and formal care practices promotes resident-orientated care, provides a good quality of life and fosters integration into the community. The following chapters in this volume discuss these issues in more detail and describe best practice in residential provision for a wide variety of client groups.

These qualities are difficult to measure yet are the essence of progressive care. Moreover, in view of the practices employed over the past 15 years in hostel wards, we believe there is still room to develop more effective care programmes.

References

Allen, H., Baigent, B., Kent, A. et al. (1993) Rehabilitation and staffing levels in a 'new look' hospital-hostel. Psychological Medicine, 23:203–11.

Bennet, D.H. (1980) The chronic psychiatric patient today. Journal of the Royal Society of Medicine, 73:301–3.

Bigelow, D.A., Cutter, D., Moore, L. et al. (1988) Characteristics of state hospital patients who are hard to place. Hospital and Community Psychiatry, 39(2):181–5.

Bridges, K., Davenport, S. and Goldberg, G. (1994) The need for hospital-based rehabilitation services. Journal of Mental Health, 3:205–12.

Cane Hill Research Team (1991) Evaluating the Closure of Cane Hill Hospital. Final Report of the Cane Hill Research Team. London, Research & Development in Psychiatry.

Dayson, D. (1993) The TAPS project 12: Crime, vagrancy, death and readmission of the long-term mentally ill during their first year of local reprovision. British Journal of Psychiatry, 162(suppl.19):40–4.

Dayson, D., Gooch, C. and Thornicroft, G. (1992) The TAPS project 16: Difficult to place long-term psychiatric patients. British Medical Journal, 305:993–5.

Garety, P.A. and Morris, I. (1984) A new unit for long-stay psychiatric patients: organization, attitudes and quality of care. Psychological Medicine, 14:183–92.

Gibbons, J.S. (1986) Care of 'new' long-stay patients in a district general psychiatric unit. Acta Psychiatrica Scandinavica, 73:582–8.

Goldberg, D.P., Bridges, K., Cooper, W. et al. (1985) Douglas House: a new type of hostel ward for chronic psychotic patients. British Journal of Psychiatry, 147:383–8.

Gooch, C. and Leff, J. (1996) The TAPS project 26: Patterns of readmission – an analysis of factors affecting the sucess of community placement. Psychological Medicine, 26:511–20.

Gudeman, J.E. and Shore, M.F. (1984) Beyond deinstitutionalization – a new class of facilities for the mentally ill. New England Journal of Medicine, 311(13):832–6.

Hallam, A. (1996) Costs and outcomes for people with special psychiatric needs. Mental Health Research Review, 3: 10–13.

Hyde, C., Bridges, K., Goldberg, D. *et al.* (1987) The evaluation of a hostel ward: a controlled study using modified cost-benefit analysis. *British Journal of Psychiatry*, **151**:805–12.

Knapp, M., Beecham, J., Hallam, A. *et al.* (1993) The TAPS project 18: The costs of community care for former long-stay psychiatric hospital residents. *Health and Social Care in the Community*, **1**(4).

Leff, J., Dayson, D. Gooch, C. *et al.* (1996) The TAPS project 19: Quality of life of long-stay patients discharged from two psychiatric institutions. *Psychiatric Services*, **47**(1):62–7.

Leff, J., Thornicroft, G., Coxhead, N. *et al.* (1994) The TAPS project 22: A five year follow-up of long-stay psychiatric patients discharged to the community. *British Journal of Psychiatry*, **165**(suppl. 25):13–17.

Lelliot, P. and Wing, J. (1994) National audit of new long-stay psychiatric patients. I: Impact on services. *British Journal of Psychiatry*, **165**:160–9.

Lelliot, P. and Wing, J. (1994) A national audit of new long-stay psychiatric patients. II: Impact on services. *British Journal of Psychiatry*, **165**:170–8.

Lewis, A. and Trieman, N. (1995) The TAPS project 29: Residential care provision in north London: a representative sample of ten facilities for mentally ill people. *International Journal of Social Psychiatry*, **41**(4):257–67.

Mann, S.A. and Cree, W. (1976) 'New long-stay' psychiatric patients: a national sample survey of fifteen mental hospitals in England and Wales. *Psychological Medicine*, **6**:603–16.

O'Driscoll, C. and Leff, J. (1993) The TAPS project 8: Design of the research study on the long-stay patients, in Leff, J. (ed.) Evaluating community placement of long-stay psychiatric patients. *British Journal of Psychiatry*, **162**(suppl.19):18–24.

Powell, R. and Hollander, D. (1994) Heading for a breakdown: crisis in admission beds. *Journal of Mental Health*, **3**:430–2.

Reda, S. (1993) The discharge of long-stay psychiatric patients into the community: a study of the patients, the staff and the public. PhD Thesis, Institute of Psychiatry, London University.

Sammut, R. (1992) Acute services study: looking at effects of changes in Bloomsbury and Islington. Presented at the seventh annual conference of the Team for the Assessment of Psychiatric Services, London, 1992.

Shepherd, G. (1995) The 'ward in a house': residential care for the severely disabled. *Community Mental Health Journal*, **31**(1):53–68.

Shepherd, G., King, C. and Fowler, D. (1994) Outcomes in hospital hostels. *Psychiatric Bulletin*, **18**:609–12.

Thomlinson, D. (1991) *Utopia, Community Care and the Retreat from the Asylums*. Milton Keynes: Open University Press.

Thornicroft, G., Margolius, O. and Jones, D. (1922) The TAPS project 6: New long-stay psychiatric patients and social deprivation. *British Journal of Psychiatry*, **161**:621–4.

Trieman, N. and Kendal, R. (1995) The TAPS project 27: After hospital: pathways patients follow in the community. *Journal of Mental Health*, **4**:423–9.

Trieman, N. and Leff, J. (1996a) The TAPS project 24: Difficult to place patients in a psychiatric hospital closure programme. *Psychological Medicine*, **26**:765–74.

Trieman, N. and Leff, J. (1996b) The TAPS project 36: Outcomes of the most difficult to place long-stay psychiatric inpatients – one year after relocation. *British Journal of Psychiatry*, **169**:289–92.

Wykes, T. and Wing, K. (1982) A ward in a house: accomodation for 'new' long-stay patients. *Acta Psychiatrica Scandinavica*, **65**:315–30.

Young, R. (ed.) (1991) *Residential Needs for Severely Disabled Psychiatric Patients – The Case for Hospital Hostels*. London, HMSO.

(A full TAPS bibliography is available from the TAPS Research Unit, 69 Fleet Road, London NW3 2QU.)

3 PUNISHMENT IN THE COMMUNITY AND THE FUTURE OF PRISON

Greg Mantle

The theme of interdependence between institutions in society is developed in this chapter in relation to the role of prisons in the criminal justice system and the purposes they serve for wider society. The critique offered in Chapter 1 of the notion of the 'total institution', and the way it has been narrowly applied to residential institutions, is further explored, and the limitations it imposes on a systemic appreciation of crime and punishment in society are exposed. In a similar vein to the previous two chapters, the conclusion reached is that the institution of prison has survived in part because it underpins the viability of community-based alternatives.

The prison remains – a stubborn presence, seemingly impervious to all attacks – and in its shadow lies 'community control'. (Cohen, 1985, p. 85)

A range of texts already exists providing accounts of, and explanations for, imprisonment and of alternative penal policies and practices. This chapter strives to make a creative contribution to this discourse. The prime proposition is that the continuing ascendancy of prison can be explained, at least in part, in terms of a widespread belief that, without it, other sentencing options available to the courts would become profoundly less viable. This belief may be true or untrue. We are unlikely ever to be in a position fully to test it out, precisely because of the power that prison commands, nevertheless, it is held widely and importantly by those who practise day to day within the penal and criminal justice system. To remove the custody card would be to bring down the rest of the deck; that is what is feared, and that is why prison will retain its particular prominence.

The thesis that prison is widely construed as the keystone of the penal system in part derives from insights gained through my probation and research work with offenders since qualification in 1978 as a front-line probation officer. I have visited many prisons within England and Wales and have always been pleased to leave them. I must admit to having experienced very similar feelings in many of the homes of offenders, captives of unemployment, inadequate education and poor accommodation. I have worked with and interviewed many offenders during and after their prison terms, and have few illusions about the brutality and degradation that prisons hand out to, mainly poor, people who have broken the law. If there was an appropriate and ready alternative, I would be very happy to embrace it. However, my conversations, reflections and study have helped me to appreciate both the importance afforded to custody in our society and the depth of concern about the effects that the demise of prison would have on the remaining penal measures.

Introduction

To say nowadays that the UK prison system is in 'crisis' normally conveys no sense of urgency and is met with little if any surprise. Prisons appear to be in a constant state of crisis: this is accepted wisdom, almost a tradition and, if propensity to riot is an acceptable indicator of crisis, unlikely to alter very much in the foreseeable future (Adams, 1994). If the slates are not being hurled by roof-top protesters, there will be an HIV/AIDS scare, a spate of tragic suicides or an escape scandal breaking across the media. How then may we understand the resilience described in Cohen's sombre words? Why are prisons still with us at all? How is it that custody, despite being in perpetual disarray and bursting at the seams, still remains in such unassailable dominance?

One response to the question is to argue that the whole penal system itself is in crisis or, indeed, that the wider criminal justice system stands at the abyss. In other words, the state of our prisons is undeniably of great concern, but so too are our probation, policing and sentencing services. The nature of that broader 'crisis' is one of legitimacy according to Cavadino and Dignan (1992), who argue that the penal system has to be 'reconstructed around the principle of respect for human rights' (p. 258). Even probation services have a good deal of ground to make up in such 'justice' terms, as probation officers struggle to switch from an organisational culture of professional autonomy towards the systematic delivery of equal opportunities within a more bureaucratic, 'managed' mode of operation (Mantle, 1995a).

The government's position is that the crisis is about overcrowding and security, hence the policies of restraining sentencers in their use of custody, building more prisons, privatisation and the introduction of security-driven regimes. Unfortunately, the rapidity and scale of policy changes with regard to the place and function of prison has been unhelpful. The 1988 Green Paper *Punishment, Custody and the Community* had unequivocally stated that imprisonment was not the most effective punishment for most crime (Home Office, 1988, 1.8), yet the present Home Secretary, Michael Howard, has vigorously promoted the catch-phrase 'Prison works', whilst simultaneously decrying the alternatives.

The purpose of prison

It has been clear to us that the prison system has not moved in any single and consistent direction during its history, but that its form and ethos have passed through a number of distinct and separate phases. (The May report, 1979, p. 7.)

What is a prison, and what is it for? Erving Goffman (1961) categorised the prison as a 'total institution', that is a place of 'residence and work where a large number of like-situated individuals, cut off from the wider society for an appreciable period of time, together lead an enclosed, formally-administered round of life'. Custodial institutions vary in terms of 'openness' or permeability of boundaries; inmates are also of varying status. Nevertheless, the prison fits Goffman's definition quite closely, and the concept is undoubtedly useful as a descriptive and analytical tool. One important spin-off is the search for 'prison' in the factory, in long-term unemployment or, for women, in the home. Unfortunately, it is all too easy to adopt the negative associations made by Goffman. The logic becomes 'Prison is a total institution and, because all total institutions are bad, prison must be bad'. Even if we accept that the total institution is, indeed, wholly bad for all inmates, we still have the issue of its worth to the community to consider. Furthermore, if the mission of prison is to punish, can it be anything other than a negative experience? Alternatively, if the purpose of prison is the containment of offenders and the concomitant protection of the community, how might the total institution as a vehicle for such policy be improved upon?

There are four key purposes of sentencing offenders: punishment, reform, deterrence and incapacitation. Prison provides an obvious punishment and a period of incapacitation. Offenders have their liberties reduced and are thus removed from their community. In terms of reform and deterrence, prison is less effective, although its deterrent effect has two dimensions: individual and general. The individual perpetrator may be deterred from committing further offences, and/or others of like mind may refrain through fear of the consequent penalty demonstrated. Prisons have traditionally been concerned, at least at the level of rhetoric, with the reform of offenders, and there remains considerable resistance to custody being seen as no more than humane confinement. A recent report by HM Chief Inspector of Prisons, Stephen Tumim (Home Office, 1993), for example, entitled *Doing Time or Using Time*, comes down firmly in favour of a role beyond the custodial. In my view, it would be far better to settle for punishment and containment as the two primary purposes of imprisonment. It is unrealistic to expect anything more: having a clear sense of purpose would be advantageous for all prison staff, and energies could be focused upon the creation of decent conditions within prisons.

Punishment implies a deliberate infliction of pain. It also usually carries an element of shame. The levels of pain and shame depend as much upon the recipient as upon the deliverer: many persistent offenders become acclimatised to the deprivations of imprisonment and even to extract a measure of kudos from 'doing bird', rather than feeling shamed by it. There are limits also to the use of 'incapacitation' as a primary purpose for custody, and various estimates of just how many people would need to be imprisoned in order to secure a significant reduction in crime have been attempted. However, a relatively few offenders account for a large slice of the total number of criminal convictions, so their incarceration will have a greater protective effect than might be at first predicted.

Arguments against prison

> Prisons do not moralize their inmates; they do not deter them from crime. (Kropotkin, 1991, p. 338.)

One yardstick of the effectiveness of prison is the rate of re-offending of ex-inmates, compared with offenders subjected to alternative, community-based sentences. There are major difficulties, however, in operationalising this type of exercise, and all findings need to be treated with considerable caution. A recent Home Office study provides an exhaustive analysis of the problems and pitfalls for the unwary; a general difficulty in this area is that official, reconviction data are only a proxy measure of re-offending:

> By no means all those offenders who, after conviction, go on to commit further crimes are caught, and not all those who are caught are convicted in court. Latest estimates from the British Crime Survey suggest that for every 100 offences committed only two result in a criminal conviction... only 50 per cent of offences are reported to the police; only 30 per cent are recorded by the police as a crime; seven per cent of crimes are cleared up; and three per cent result in a caution or conviction. (Lloyd *et al.*, 1994, p. 5.)

The fact that 97 per cent of criminal offences result in neither a caution nor a conviction is an important counterpoint to crude claims for the reductivist efficacy of custody. However, it is an equally pertinent caveat for assertions about the similar achievements of non-custodial measures. To discover that custody has no or little effect upon the likelihood of re-offending is a matter of some concern, but critics take things a step further in arguing that custody actually increases the probability of further transgressions. The idea that custodial institutions act as 'schools of crime', wherein the skills and underpinning attitudes of criminal activity are cascaded, honed and amplified, is a powerful one and likely to have application in many cases, although gauging the scale of such an effect would be very difficult. Furthermore, there are many alternative opportunities for learning about crime and, indeed, for fostering a resentment of legitimate authority. I am thinking here not only of informal, neighbourhood networks in our inner cities and on our 'sink' estates, but also of the institutionalised grouping together of offenders as an adjunct to bail and, post-sentence, as an integral component of their probation or community service programmes. Offenders are routinely clustered in probation and bail hostels. Group work is already the norm for probation programme centres, and, as budgetary cuts continue to bite, probation managers are looking much more favourably at the cost savings to be had from group rather than traditional, individual supervision for probationers. Offenders subject to community service orders also spend much of their work time together, and opportunities will no doubt exist within these periods or later for criminogenic liaison.

A further posited effect of custody is that of 'brutalisation'. Offenders are treated so badly that they leave custodial institutions in a much worse condition than at their point of entry into the system. There are two threads in the argument: first, that damage is done by the very act of containment itself, and second, that the nature of the regime, environment or culture within the institution brutalises the offender. Proponents of the former would object to custody even if containment conditions were made as humane as possible, whilst a more reformist ideology is characteristically associated with the latter assertion. There are strong ethical grounds for minimising any harm done to inmates by their incarceration, and returning offenders to the community even less able to live without resorting to crime than they previously were is inherently contradictory. The Woolf Report (1991), champions the notion of a 'community prison', the main advantage of which would be to help maintain the links between inmates and their families during the custodial period, aiding the subsequent process of resettlement.

Most people serving custodial sentences are young, lower-class males, and a high proportion of them are from ethnic minorities. In 1992 about one-quarter of the sentenced population was aged 21–24 years (Home Office, 1994b, para. 1.20). On 30 June 1992 about 15 per cent of males and an astonishing 26 per cent of females in Prison Service establishments were of ethnic minority origin, while 10 per cent of males and 20 per cent of females were of West Indian/Guyanese or African origin (Home Office, 1994a, 1.22). By comparing these proportions with the corresponding figures for the population of England and Wales as a whole, and then accounting for the uneven spread over social class divisions, it is possible to conclude that far too many black people end up in custody. Their experiences of racism within our custodial institutions are well documented (Genders and Player, 1989). Many prisoners are mentally ill, illiterate, homeless, alcoholic or addicted to drugs, and the under-resourcing of community care has served to exacerbate an already appalling situation. The evidence in support of a contention that the 'wrong people' are treated custodially is weighty and hard to refute. Just who the 'right people' might be is an interesting question, but, presumably, they would include many of the offenders responsible for the vast amount of crime unrecorded, undetected and unpoliced. The shape, rather than the size, of the prison population might therefore be subject to change.

The number of people incarcerated in England and Wales at any one point in time is rarely not a subject of considerable concern. The number of offenders sentenced to immediate (i.e. unsuspended) custody for all offence types increased sharply from 1993 to 1994, from 58,400 to a figure of 69,200. Within this total, some 52,400 offenders aged 21 years and above had been sent to prisons and 16,800 offenders aged 14–20 years had been sent to young offender institutions (Home Office, 1995, Table 7A). These figures may appear high, but it is worth comparing them with the respective statistic for 1985, when a peak total of 83,300 offenders were sentenced to immediate custody. The proportionate use of unsuspended custody is, in fact, lower now than it was in 1987: 18.4 per cent in 1987 compared with 17.1 per cent in 1994 (Home Office, 1995, Table 7.15). Of course, the size of the prison population is affected by a much wider set of variables, including the length of sentences, arrangements for early release and the numbers on remand awaiting trial or sentence. With regard to the length of sentences, the proportion of long sentences has more than doubled in the period from 1984 to 1992 (Home Office, 1994a, 1.19), whilst changes to remission for short-sentence prisoners in August 1987 reduced the population by 3,000 (Home Office, 1994a, 1.10). The remand population in 1992 was 10,100, a steep increase on the 1982 figure of 7,400, while the size of the sentenced population actually decreased slightly (Home Office, 1994a, 1.13).

A final and related criticism is that, compared with many other countries, the prison population *per capita* of England and Wales is too high. However, our record is by no means the worst and compares very favourably with, for example, the USA, where the rate is some four times higher. There are weaknesses too in making a comparison solely on the basis of population. Countries have very different crime rates, for example, and constructing a league table based on the prison population per recorded crime places England and Wales much closer to the bottom. This is not to advocate complacency but simply to sound a cautionary note; the factors that may contribute to a 'high' prison population are worthy of meticulous scrutiny. Custody is a costly resource and should be avoided if at all possible. Nevertheless, there needs to be a balance struck between these considerations and the need to punish offenders and to protect the public from their activities.

A world without prison

The idea of a penal landscape that did not include 'prison' is certainly beyond most people's ken. Pointing (1986, p. 1) describes support for custody as a 'deeply-held emotional force' and prison as the 'symbolic core of the criminal justice system' (p. 2). He argues that the space for 'alternatives to custody' will always be shaped by the emotional/moral dimension of public support for prison. The signification of community-based court disposals as 'alternatives' was itself a reflection and reproduction of prisons' ideological dominance.

A hallmark of the carceral society is that its members find it difficult to conceive of a penal system lacking imprisonment as the ultimate back-up to every type of penalty... Most probably a very small minority of offenders would stubbornly resist all attempts to regulate them. Unless they went on to commit very serious crimes we would just have to put up with their anti-social behaviour. (Carlen, 1990, p. 124)

Carlen proposes the abolition of women's imprisonment, with the exception of a small number of prison places for those convicted or accused of the most serious crimes, such as murder or terrorism. Her concomitant strategic aims are to: (1) expand the use of community service and probation orders; (2) enhance compliance with community sentences by making them more attractive to offenders; and (3) increase the feasibility of sentences. Offenders who did decide not to comply with their court order would thus be free to do so; there would simply be too few of them to worry about. Should they continue to offend, they would then be allowed to do so; there would again only be a few such cases and their further offending would anyway not be 'serious'. The primary weaknesses in Carlen's position are, first, that it fails to acknowledge the seriousness of offences such as robbery, drug trafficking and domestic burglary, and second, that it ignores the need to protect already disadvantaged communities from the activities of criminals. The presumption that citizens should, and indeed would, be willing to accept such continuing predation at the hands of convicted offenders is highly suspect.

Very few people would argue for the total abolition of custody as there is a widespread belief that prison will always be required for the deserving few:

By their actions some men and a few women in all societies forfeit their right to their liberty. Prisons will always be needed for the small number of human beings who cannot control their aggression and who behave violently towards others, or whose uncontrollable greed undermines the society in which they operate. (Blackstone, 1990, p. 54)

Unfortunately, the number of potential candidates for custody before or after sentence is actually rather large. For example, in 1994, a total of 37,600 offenders were sentenced for indictable offences of violence against the person, a further 4,500 for sexual offences, 4,900 for robbery and 38,000 for burglary (Home Office, 1995, Table 7.2). Another way of approaching the issue of quantification is to reflect on the fact that about 34 per cent of men born in 1953 had been convicted of a standard list offence by the age of 40 (Home Office, 1995, 1.20). Blackstone perhaps underestimates the number of men who at some point in their lives will not (rather than 'cannot') control their aggression and require humane confinement in order to secure the protection of the public. Custody is a feature both of judicial process and of judicial punishment. In other words, society uses custodial institutions for those accused of crimes who are denied bail and for those who have been convicted and sentenced. Any argument for the abandonment of confinement must satisfactorily address the loss of these two key functions. Given that the prison population of England and Wales, at 51,678, reached its highest ever point in March 1995 (*Independent*, 31 May 1995, p. 19), the strain placed upon community-based alternatives would be considerable.

Alternatives to prison: a story of lost opportunities

At no other time in British penal history has the use of imprisonment been under such sustained criticism. The time is ripe, so it would seem, for a major penal initiative to promote non-custodial alternatives. (Willis, 1986, p. 18)

Ten years after Willis' bold pronouncement, the bag is a mixed one. The use of immediate and suspended custody has indeed lessened, and the use of community sentences has undoubtedly increased. However, the degree of displacement is arguably not as great as might have been expected, given the range of new penalties made available to the courts and given the efforts expended (1) to make community sentences more attractive to sentencers, and (2) to introduce criteria for the employment of custodial measures, in effect to tie the hands of sentencers. There are pitfalls in this kind of analysis. Attending to only some of the disposals available can lead to distortions. In an important sense, many sentences constitute 'alternatives to custody' simply because they are available, and, with this in mind, the wider range of penalties that might be seen as displacing custody is now examined.

Fines

Most people sentenced in the courts of England and Wales are fined. In 1994 a fine was imposed upon 75 per cent of the 1,407,100 offenders dealt with (Home Office, 1995, 7.6). It is most often used by sentencers for summary (less serious) matters, and fines represent about eight out of every ten sentences handed down by magistrates. For both summary and indictable offences, the use of the fine has dropped quite steeply over the past decade. The percentage of offenders fined for indictable offences fell from 40 per cent in 1989 to 31 per cent in 1994 (Home Office, 1995, 7.9). Because the fine is mainly utilised for less serious offences, its place as an alternative to custody is questionable. It would be reasonable to argue that most offenders who are fined are also unlikely to be imprisoned. During 1994 more than 22,700 people were gaoled for default, most for failing to pay fines for motoring offences or theft, many for TV licence evasion or for non-payment of community charge (Penal Affairs Consortium, 1995, p. 17). There is a further factor that undermines any attempt to construe the fine as an alternative to custody. Failure to pay is itself sanctioned by imprisonment, and non-payment of fines in fact accounts for about 20 per cent of all prison receptions of sentenced offenders (the distinction here being with people remanded in custody, awaiting trial or sentence). Because the average length of stay is no more than a few days, fine defaulters constitute only a very small proportion of the prison population at any one time, although they do have a disproportionately high impact on prison procedures.

The problem of what to do about fine default has long been recognised, whilst satisfactory solutions have remained singularly elusive. In 1970 the Advisory Council on the Penal System recommended that defaulters who failed to pay solely because they lacked the means to do so should not be committed to prison. Numerous studies have since demonstrated that having insufficient funds is a key reason for non-payment, so how is it that prison receptions for default continue unabated? The legitimacy of changing policy is clearly hard to refute, and there are plenty of alternatives to pursue, such as imposing a short community service order. My argument is that these options have not found favour because, without the ultimate sanction of custody, they are perceived as having little chance of success. This belief is sometimes visible in the most unexpected places, for example:

> One fundamental question remains: should imprisonment be retained at all as a sanction for fine default? To begin to answer this it is important to acknowledge that... a small minority of imprisoned fine defaulters do wilfully refuse to pay. Perhaps a rather larger number only pay up because of the threat posed by a committal warrant. (Prison Reform Trust, 1989, p. 39)

The suggestion here is that, given the chance of impunity, many offenders would avoid paying their fines, and, in the absence of prison, offenders would indeed have little to fear. Studies of fine default might usefully address the central question of why people do pay rather than restricting attention to why they do not. Looking back over a longer time span, the proportionate use of the fine for adult indictable offenders decreased from 55 per cent in 1975 to 53 per cent in 1980 and to 41 per cent in 1989 (Cavadino and Dignan, 1992, Table 7.1). So, even in the case of more serious offences, courts have relied heavily upon the use of financial penalties and, as such, fines must play a significant part in the displacement of custodial measures. The decline in usage might therefore suggest an increase in custodial sentencing; to some degree, this is likely to be true. However, variations in the use of other sentences are perhaps more significant, and to such we now attend.

Community service

The term 'community sentence' is used to signify probation, community service, combination, supervision and attendance centre orders. A total of 129,000 community sentences were given by courts in England and Wales in 1994, marking a rise of 12 per cent over the previous year. Most of this increase was accounted for by rises in the numbers of probation and combination orders. In 1994 28 per cent of offenders received a community sentence, a figure that has increased annually since the 1989 rate of 20 per cent (Home Office, 1995, 7.9).The proportionate use of community service for indictable (more serious) offences has risen steadily each year, from 7 per cent in 1989 to 10–11 per cent in 1993 and 1994, whilst the use of the probation order has stayed at 10–11 per cent over this period (Home Office, 1995, Table 7.3).

The community service order is a much more recent addition to the court's sanctions than is probation. Following its experimental introduction under the Criminal Justice Act 1972, it became available to the courts on a national basis in 1975 and quickly became firmly established. In 1994 a total of 49,500 community service orders were made, a rise of 3 per cent over 1993 and nearly matching the use of probation. However, in the Crown Court, the use of community service actually fell in 1993–94 from 12,200 to 11,000, whilst the fall in the number of probation orders over the same period was much less. Since October 1992 it has been possible for courts to combine community service and probation elements within a 'combination order'. This has quickly proved to be popular with sentencers, and in 1994 some 12,400 orders were made (Home Office, 1995, Table 7.1).

Community service owes much of its popularity with sentencers to its essentially punitive nature. Offenders are required to undertake unpaid work, usually of a manual type, ostensibly on behalf of the community, and they do this within a proscribed period of 40–240 hours. Stringent national standards were introduced by the Government in 1989 in an attempt to amplify the use of community service as an alternative to custody. Any assessment of the success of the community service order as a displacement for custody would need to examine the risk of custody at point of sentence and the likelihood of breach, revocation and custodial re-sentencing. It is fair to say that many shorter community service orders have been alternatives to a fine rather than custody. The momentum for sentencers to employ community service in this way is unsurprising given that most people appearing before the criminal courts are already impoverished and likely to experience considerable difficulty in paying pecuniary penalties. In cases of failure to comply with the order, a court may simply take no action, punish the breach, allowing the order to continue, or revoke the order and re-sentence the offender. Many orders are revoked, and, of these, the proportion dealt with by way of immediate custody is relatively high, of the order of 30 per cent (Home Office, 1991, 7.22). A significant question mark must therefore be raised concerning the validity of claims for community service as a displacement for custody. In many cases, the order may, in fact, be providing an additional route into prisons or young offender institutions.

Probation

The probation order has been with us since the 1907 Probation of Offenders Act and, for much of the century, has provided one of the main 'alternatives' to custody. Until the implementation of the Criminal Justice Act 1991, probation had technically been an alternative to sentence rather than to custody. Courts were able to release the offender without sentencing, by placing him or her under the supervision of a probation officer for a period of between 6 months and 3 years. The 1991 Act remoulded probation as a sentence of the court, alongside and available for combination with the other community disposals.

The aims of probation are defined as:

- securing the rehabilitation of the offender;
- protecting the public from harm from the offender; or
- preventing the offender from committing further offences.

(Powers of Criminal Courts Act 1973, s.2(1), substituted by s.8(1) of
the Criminal Justice Act 1991.)

Sentencers are able to include a range of extra requirements in
probation orders, making the disposal appropriate for offences of
varying levels of seriousness and for offenders with a wide spread of
problems. In cases where the risk of custody is highest, it is possible to
make a single 'combination order' including elements of community
service and probation supervision. The probation element might also
embrace a number of special conditions, such as attendance at a
Probation Programme Centre, offering group work addressing motor
vehicle-related crime or alcohol abuse. Even residential or medical
treatment requirements may be stipulated by the courts, making
probation the most flexible disposal available to sentencers. The gulf in
terms of deprivation of liberty between a 6 months order, without
extra conditions, and a 3 years term of supervision, including a residential requirement, is vast and suggests that probation should hardly
be short of currency in the courts. Despite this enormous potential,
the probation order has enjoyed variable success since the Second
World War.

During its early years, probation had a significant impact upon
custodial sentencing and accounted for about one-third of all
indictable offenders sentenced immediately prior to the outbreak of
war. There followed a steady decline to a low point in the mid-1970s
and a subsequent resurgence. The number of probation orders made
by all courts in 1994 was 50,500, a sharp increase on the previous
year, although the proportionate use of probation for indictable
offences has remained at about 10–11 per cent over the period
1989–94. In the Crown Court, however, the proportionate usage
dipped from nearly 15 per cent to less than 13 per cent over the period
1993–94 (Home Office, 1995, Table 7.1), suggesting that the attrac-
tion of probation may be waning within the key 'custody crucible'
despite the government's earlier attempts to boost its currency through
the introduction of a comprehensive set of national standards. Only a
tiny fraction of probation orders are terminated for failure to comply
with requirements, and this proportion has stayed remarkably
constant over recent years despite radical shifts in the nature of probation work and in the statutory and policy frames within which the
order is situated. Of the 43,430 probation orders terminating in 1985,
only 2 per cent were for failure to comply; the respective figure for the
43,772 finishers in 1993 is 3 per cent (Home Office 1994b, Table
2.10). The number of terminations in which a further offence has been

committed is much larger, of the order of 10–15 per cent. However, about 80 per cent of probation orders are either completed early 'for good progress' or run their full course. Probation officers would no doubt wish to argue that they are now dealing with more serious offenders and therefore that the risk of failure has grown. On the other hand, the average length of probation orders has decreased over the past decade, in effect reducing the likelihood of an early, ignominious denouement.

Recent evidence from a survey of ex-probationers (Mantle, 1995b) highlights the significance of prospective imprisonment in offender responses to community supervision. Participants were asked to identify the likely results of committing offences within the currency of their probation order: about two-thirds replied 'prison' and only 3 per cent played down the seriousness of such a scenario. Given this widespread belief amongst probationers, it seems reasonable to suppose that their present high levels of compliance might be forfeited should the underpinning threat of custody be removed.

Attendance centre

> For all the rhetoric, senior attendance centres do not seem on any measure to be acting to any marked degree as an alternative to custody. (Mair, 1991, p. 190)

In cases when an offence is punishable by imprisonment, anyone aged less than 21 years may be made the subject of an attendance centre order. The order can also be made for non-compliance with other community sentences and for fine default. Attendance centres are usually run by police officers and offer a package of physical training and instruction on various topics and activities such as first aid, craft work and citizenship. The offender is required to attend on Saturdays, for 2 or 3 hour periods depending on their age. The primary aim of an attendance centre order is to punish through deprivation of leisure time, and centres have been seen as an appropriate way of dealing with juvenile and young adult 'football hooligans'. Failure to comply can result in a return to court, where the offender may be dealt with by means of a custodial sentence or by other means.

Prior to the arrival of the Criminal Justice Act 1991, the attendance centre order had, at least in theory, constituted an alternative to a short custodial sentence. Its redefined status, alongside other disposals such as probation and community service, is, as a sentence in its own right, to be employed for offences of a seriousness considered to be below the custody threshold. Because of the variability of sentencing practice, however, it is reasonable to argue that the attendance centre order could still act as an alternative to custody. What remains clear, however, is that the attendance centre order has had little real impact as a displacement of custody. It is very rarely used in the Crown Court, which is where the proportionate use of custody is highest. In 1994, of 71,000 offenders sentenced in the Crown Court, 7,300 young offender institution orders were made, compared with only some 100 attendance centre orders. The respective figures for Magistrates' Courts are 1,336,000 offenders sentenced, 9,600 sent to young offender institutions and 7,200 sent to attendance centres (Home Office, 1995, Table 7.1). The proportionate use of the attendance centre order has remained at about 0.5 per cent during the period 1988–94. In contrast, the use of the community service order for all offences has increased from 2.3 per cent in 1988 to 3.5 per cent in 1994 (Home Office, 1995, Table 7A).

The suspended prison sentence

The fully suspended sentence of imprisonment is the most direct alternative to immediate custody available to the courts. It was introduced by the Criminal Justice Act 1967 as a remedy for the rising prison population, despite a great deal of contemporaneous controversy about its likely effectiveness. Where the court decides that an offence is so serious that only a custodial sentence (of not more than 2 years duration) can be justified, it may suspend the sentence for an 'operational' period of between 1 and 2 years. In the Crown Court, a suspended sentence supervision order may be added, requiring the offender to be supervised by a probation officer. However, the suspended sentence of imprisonment is normally characterised by minimal external intervention and deprivation of liberty, providing the subject does not reoffend within the operational lifetime of the order (Mantle and Swinden, 1991). Should an offence be committed, the likelihood of custody is high, and, for this reason, suspended sentences have been portrayed as contributing to the ever-burgeoning prison population rather than as displacing custody. They have also been inappropriately used by sentencers in cases in which probation or community service, rather than custody, would have been expected.

In spite of its popularity with sentencers, the suspended sentence has found little favour with the present government. The measure has not fitted in with the 'just desserts' sentencing framework introduced by the Criminal Justice Act 1991, and its use has consequently tumbled from 22,000 in 1992 to 3,800 in 1993 and to just 3,200 in 1994 (Home Office, 1995, Table 7.1). In the Crown Court, the fall was from 16 per cent in the first three-quarters of 1992 to 6 per cent in the last quarter and 2–3 per cent in the last three-quarters of 1993 and throughout 1994. The 1991 Act also removed the partly suspended sentence of imprisonment from the list of available court's disposal, although the order had been little used since its introduction in 1982.

The longer-term effects, if any, of this demise of the suspended sentence of imprisonment are difficult to predict. Perhaps the most significant lesson to be derived from the brief but eventful history of the 'bender', as it is commonly called, is that policies aimed at displacing custody are not readily translated into practice. It is also important to recognise that such well-meaning attempts to reduce the prison population may, paradoxically, have the reverse effect. However, the key design fault in the suspended sentence is the enthusiasm it appears to promote in sentencers in England and Wales to deal with breaches of the order by way of an immediate custodial penalty. There is no reason in principle why this should be so, and indeed other juris-dictions have successfully employed the suspended sentence to reduce their prison populations (Rutherford, 1986, p. 159). This is not to argue that the suspended sentence of imprisonment could be viable without the risk of its implementation in cases of breach: it is the degree of risk that is being questioned.

Conclusion: understanding prison's survival

Stanley and Baginsky (1984, p. 9) assert that prison has survived for three reasons: inertia, the philosophy of treatment and because it seems to be needed. On the basis of our earlier review of the main non-custodial sentences, it is possible to add a fourth reason, namely that alternative measures have had a limited displacement effect. The authors identify 'inertia' as the most important of the three factors: they point to the reluctance of sentencers to change their practices, to the role played by public attitudes to crime and punishment, and to the insulated momentum of the prison system. Their analysis is not wholly convincing. It suggests that all resistance to change is irra-tional, which is simply not true. In addition, the significance of the belief that prison is needed appears to be underestimated. That need is essentially threefold: first, as a punishment and containment; second, as an element of judicial process; and third, as a way of ensuring the viability of other sentences. My contention is that this third aspect of how the importance of prison is construed has not been afforded the recognition it deserves.

References

Adams, R. (1994) *Prison Riots in Britain and the USA*. London, Macmillan.
Advisory Council on the Penal System (1970) *Non-custodial and Semi-custodial Penalties*. London, HMSO.
Blackstone, T. (1990) *Prisons and Penal Reform*. London, Chatto & Windus.
Carlen, P. (1990) *Alternatives to Women's Imprisonment*. Milton Keynes, Open University Press.
Cavadino, M. and Dignan, J. (1992) *The Penal System: An Introduction*. London, Sage.
Cohen, S. (1985) *Visions of Social Control*. Cambridge, Polity Press.
Committee of Inquiry into the United Kingdom Prison Services (1979) (The May report) Cmnd 7673. London, HMSO.
Genders, E. and Player, E. (1989) *Race Relations in Prisons*. Oxford, Clarendon Press.
Goffman, E. (1961) *Asylums*. New York, Doubleday Anchor Books.
Home Office (1988) *Punishment, Custody and the Community*, Cmnd 424. London, HMSO.
Home Office (1991) *The Sentence of the Court*. London, HMSO.
Home Office (1993) *Report of a Review by Her Majesty's Chief Inspector of Prisons for England and Wales*, Cmnd 2128. London, HMSO.
Home Office (1994a) *Prison Statistics: England and Wales, 1992*. London, HMSO.
Home Office (1994b) *Probation Statistics: England and Wales, 1993*. London, HMSO.
Home Office (1995) *Criminal Statistics: England and Wales, 1994*. London, HMSO.
Kropotkin, P. (1991) *In Russian and French Prisons*. Montreal, Black Rose Books.
Lloyd, C., Mair, G. and Hough, M. (1994) *Explaining Reconviction Rates; A Critical Analysis*. Home Office Research Study 136. London, HMSO.
Mair, G. (1991) *Part-time Punishment: The Origins and Development of Senior Attendance Centres*. London, HMSO.
Mantle, G. (1995a) *Probation Work with Offenders: Recipients' Perspectives: Report to Essex Probation Service*. Chelmsford, Anglia Polytechnic University.
Mantle, G. (1995b) Probation: offenders have their say. *Justice of the Peace and Local Government Law*, **159**(22):368–9.
Mantle, G. and Swinden, D. (1991) Recommending suspended sentences. *Probation Journal*, **38**(4):190–2.
Penal Affairs Consortium (1995), in *Guardian*, 17 July, 1995.
Pointing, J. (ed.) (1986) *Alternatives to Custody*. Oxford, Blackwell.

Prison Reform Trust (1989) *Tackling Fine Default*. London, Prison Reform Trust.

Rutherford, A. (1986) *Prisons and the Process of Justice*. Oxford, Oxford University Press.

Stanley, S. and Baginsky, M. (1984) *Alternatives to Prison: An Examination of Non-custodial Sentencing of Offenders*. London, Peter Owen.

Willis, A. (1986) Alternatives to imprisonment: an elusive paradise?, in Pointing, J. (ed.) *Alternatives to Custody*. Oxford, Blackwell, pp. 162–82.

Woolf, Rt. Hon. Lord Justice H. and Tumim, His Hon. Judge S. (1991) *Prison Disturbances April 1990: Report of an Inquiry*, Cmnd 1456. London, HMSO.

4 SHELTER-WITH-CARE AND THE COMMUNITY CARE REFORMS – NOTES ON THE EVOLUTION OF ESSENTIAL SPECIES

Bleddyn Davies

The potential role of various forms of residential care – 'shelter-with-care' – for elderly people and people with disabilities is the subject of this chapter. The blurring of the boundaries between residential and community-based services in the most innovatory forms of community care is described and the inhibiting effect on such developments of the narrow dualistic conception of residential care within communities acknowledged. Professor Davies' chapter forges a link between the critique of dualistic conceptions of how communities care, made in earlier chapters, and the accounts which follow of the diversity of roles that good-quality residential facilities can play in promoting community care. The conclusion is that reform of community care in the UK, far from sounding the death knell of residential institutions, provides opportunities for their more complete integration into caring communities.

Bruce Vladeck wrote that the American nursing home was like the story of the mule in the settlement of the West. Without it, the history would have been different. However, it was simply not the main focus for anyone, certainly not for those living through it. An exaggeration perhaps. But during the years of reform, 'shelter-with-care' (SWC) has

71

received perhaps less attention in the British community care reforms than did nursing homes in Lyndon Johnson's introduction of Medicare and Medicaid. The reforms could provide a context that could evolve an even nobler family of beasts, not one or two species but several, all drawing genes from the same British SWC stock. This chapter speculates on how that will happen and on some of the pressures on the evolution influencing the kind of beasts they will be.

Several propositions will be discussed.

1.   *Because the most attention-attracting emphasis of the health and community care reforms was to make the policy institutions more 'self-inventing'* (Klein, 1995), *attention was (deliberately or otherwise) distracted from national policy interventions to develop individual services.* Klein argues that the British have made the institutions of social policy 'self-inventing' – that is incentives have been created to respond in the specification of ends and means to uncertainty, turbulence and long-term change in the environment – as an accidental result of the Thatcher administration's development of markets for the allocation of resources in public policy. The argument will be elaborated in order to provide the assumptions for the prediction of the character of new species. The elaboration is one perspective on the nature of the reforms.

2.   *It is in the nature of the reformed structures, with their creation of markets giving incentives to organisational adjustment to the environment, that each service supplied will be more formed than previously by a whole range of 'substitutes' and 'complements'.* One aspect of the reforms is of strategic importance for this mutual influence. The reforms are aimed at providing a choice of home care for more users. The degree to which this is accomplished will influence the demand for, and hence the role and nature of, SWC. There is some early but important evidence about changes in the nature of the roles and nature of home care. Likewise, there is evidence about the implications surrounding who will demand SWC. Some of that evidence will be discussed below.

3.   *We should broaden and deepen the understanding of development overseas to help to translate the values reflected in the reforms into working models of SWC, so that the broadening and deepening may require government to stimulate the collation and dissemination of that information and argument.* A section below illustrates overseas models and develops a typology that can partially

replace the classifications based broadly on a 'continuum of care' excessively focused on a classification of modes of care founded on 'dependency'.

4. *Do the new 'self-inventing' policy structures ensure the optimal collation and dissemination of information in SWC?* Only in the most unlikely of circumstances do markets yield the most equitable distributions with the greatest economic efficiency. Indeed, it might almost be said that in most advanced economies, whenever there is a market, there is almost certainly a trade and industry policy of sorts to correct the market failures. The provision of information and the stimulation of analysis are among the most common trade and industry policies. We ask whether policy intervention is needed to disseminate new ideas about how to provide SWC that combines good care with the conferment on residents of status, rights and feelings of maximum feasible autonomy. The British can, with benefit, learn from developments elsewhere – useful practical 'technological' innovations intended to reduce the demands on human help or make its effort more effective, in organisational features and artefacts for delivering the care component in various contexts. That will also be discussed below.

The reforms as the creation of self-inventing institutions

The focus of the reforms, the most radical and coherent national effort in the modernisation of community and long-term care anywhere in the world, has been the structuring of the system, the promotion of values and priorities, setting goals and establishing the machinery and processes for achieving them. They are about setting frameworks to mediate the demand for care services and their nature and content.

Traditional service focus of policy

The new focus contrasts both with pre-reform UK policy and with the balance of the content of reforms in most other countries.

Service focus in reforms overseas

In the USA, the most publicised element of the Clinton plan for long-term care reform was the development of the financing mechanism, although the sophisticated American argument has linked financing reform firmly with improving equity, effectiveness and efficiency in the supply of care in a way which has not yet generally been done in the UK. Despite the attention to financing mechanisms, the federal government has provided financial inducements to develop home care and directly subsidises the payment of nursing home fees of the poor through the Medicaid programme. (Nursing homes continue to dominate the flow of funds: only 36 per cent of government long-term care expenditures for elderly people were for home care services: Wiener *et al.*, 1994). The Medicaid subsidisation of the poor is accompanied by complex regulation of inputs and process, particularly in nursing homes. On every conceivable question about their SWC, the Americans have produced research literature that is vast by the standards of the UK and other countries generally. Some examples are the large numbers of texts on care provision and the use of techniques for managers and care workers; the analyses showing the strengths and weakness of care; the analyses of the impact of regulative devices on indicators of the quality of life and care; many analyses of the patterns of utilisation of services through time and influences on them, and the dependence of the demand for some services on the supply of others; and the studies of the evolution of demand and supply of care in the very long run. The federal and state governments sponsor publicly usable databases that give a richness of information which we can only envy. One can deny neither the wealth of the analysis of services nor indeed the direct sponsorship of the development of variety of specific services in the USA.

In Australia, too, the Aged Care Reform Strategy has mixed inducements to develop particular services and needs-based planning of the balance of care with target levels of provision of the main kinds of service. Indeed, some of the devices used by the Australian commonwealth government could have stepped straight out of British history immediately prior to the oil crisis. It has been suggested that the interest in the substance of service policy mirrored the equity concerns of Labour administration of the 1980s reflected in the Social Justice Strategy (Howe, 1996).

In these countries, the logic underlying many of the components of reform packages has been directed both at specific services and at ensuring access for those in need, and at other commissioning issues.

During the initial stage of the UK reforms, the focus has, in contrast, consistently been on creating structures for service commissioning despite – as Klein predicts to be the consequence of grafting market mechanisms onto hierarchical and politically sensitive organisation – switches of emphasis in central government priorities for the development of community care, a lack of pressure to develop some of the components originally perceived to be essential, and the introduction of new pressures, exacerbated at the local level by incrementalist and slow changes (Davies *et al.*, 1996; Gostick *et al.*, in press).

Service focus in UK policy history

The international differences are less striking than the contrast with earlier epochs in the post-war history of care. First, the post-war reform itself was primarily about the provision of services. Second, whereas the emphasis of the current reforms is to provide the choice of staying at home for more of those in need of care, the post-war emphasis was on SWC, more specifically on the residential home. The concept of the local authority residential home run by the new local authority welfare departments replaced the workhouse run by the public assistance committees.

The Bevanite concept was of the private residential hotel, allowing a sense of independence and self-respect, residents having personal possessions, mostly single rooms, near friends: 'there is no reason at all why the public character of these places should not be very much in the background, because the whole idea is that the welfare authorities should provide them and charge an economic rent for them, so that any old persons who wished to go there may get there, in exactly the same way as many well-to-do people have been accustomed to go into residential hotels' (*Hansard*, 1948, vol. 444).

The thinking turned out to have been confused. The potential increase in supply was underestimated, but there were reasons that reflected processes common to other contexts and other countries, ones whose implication we shall refer to again later. There was a waiting list for chronic sick beds equal to one-sixth of their number and therefore diversion of demand to residential care. Also, those admitted became increasingly handicapped. (It was estimated that 15 per cent of the residents in 1950 were still there in 1959, and that coping with survivors among successive waves of long-lived entrants would have required a rate of increase in provision slightly larger than the rate of increase needed to cope with each new wave of community entrants: Davies, 1968; Davies *et al.*, 1973) First priority was given to those less able to perform acts of daily living in allocating the places. Thus Bevan's concept of the appropriate target group proved unrealistic: 'the types of people who are still able to look afer themselves... "do for themselves", but who are unable to do the housework, the laundry, cook meals and things of that sort'; that is persons with difficulties with the instrumental but not the personal care tasks of daily living, those who, decades later but prior to the current reforms, had become the higher priority clientele of the home care services (*Hansard*, 1948, col. 1609).

There were critics. Again, their basic arguments and suggestions are still made, although in forms which reflect the accumulation of experience and the elaboration of ideas. Alderman Messer, Chairman of the National Old People's Welfare Committee (later Age Concern England), disagreed about targeting. He argued that elderly people should not enter residential homes as long as they could manage in their own homes and that domiciliary services should be more highly developed for that purpose (*Hansard*, 1948, col. 16). Alice Bacon, a social security minister in the 1960s, argued for the building of housing suitable for elderly persons. History proved Messer to be have been right and Bevan wrong – although those were busy times for Bevan, and many could have said, with Bessy Braddock: 'I think of what we are repealing more than of what we are proposing' (*Hansard*, 1948, col. 1615).

In the UK, at least, the emphasis was on the virtues of the home rather than the nursing facility, and the adaptation (such as the Circular of 1955 permitting larger homes to cope with the greater disability) retained that model. We shall see below how some of the progressive American states shifted from nursing homes as health-related facilities to new forms of SWC, some of which were not unlike British residential homes. The opposite happened in France and the USA, with far worse consequences. In France, the increasing pressure of those needing personal care led to the introduction of a specifically medico-health care model, with the development during the 1970s of medium- and long-stay wards and medical care sections in old people's homes (Pous *et al.*, 1992). The consequence was an overlap of the range of disabilities of the social and health forms of SWC, with a deepening of the gulf between the agencies, exacerbated by the decentralisation policy that made one the responsibility of the *département* and the other the responsibility of the *région* (Pous *et al.*, 1992). In the USA, Lyndon Johnson's introduction of Medicaid provided a financing mechanism and regulation for the nursing home as a medicalised organisation, destroyed the less medicalised 'mom-and-pop' homes and established regulations and a financing mechanism that inhibited the development of SWC alternatives for more than 20 years in all but a few renegade states. In the UK, in contrast, there was a slow diversion of the role of nursing homes from a general, often short-stay function, to their role in long-term care of the elderly. Given the current age distribution of patients, it is surprising that only 70 per cent of residents were elderly by 1983 (Challis and Bartlett, 1987). Indeed, it was only from the mid-1980s that the increase in the number of places in them accelerated quickly compared with that in independent residential homes, reflecting the acceleration of change in the role of the hospital (Audit Commission, 1992).

From the late 1950s, as the boom in the local authority creation of family housing waned, authorities' technostructure was progressively applied to housing for special groups. However, the relevant central government applied the same service supply focus. Policy sponsorship of new models for the delivery of care into elderly people's housing was inhibited by that and other factors: the Department of Health focus on residential care, the division of labour between health and housing ministries at the central government level and the unimportance to the Department of Environment of housing for frail elderly people needing close supervision and personal care packages. The gap between social services and housing in many local authorities has always been narrower than in the central government, and there has been a strong trend in urban authorities to create departments spanning housing and social services, as the central government's discouragement of that arrangement diminished. At no time was there the merger of community services, housing and health at central government level that there was at the Australian commonwealth level.

Ineffectiveness of the old service focus

Although the lead agencies at national and local levels were primarily service focused, development was slow and produced little variety in provision. The balance of the portfolio of work of the Social Work Service of the Department of Health and Social Security (DHSS; replaced by the Social Services Inspectorate in response to the Financial Management Initiative during the mid-1980s) was quite unrelated to the relative scale of service operations, the spending level, the potential for improving cost-effectiveness or even the effectiveness of client numbers in recipient groups. Middle managers in social services departments focused insufficiently on outcomes, and most were unaware of new models and arguments from other countries. One may ask whether some of the scandalous failures in SWC institutions, for the elderly as well as for other groups, would still have been happening had it been a golden age. The learning was mainly inductive. There was not the clear ethic, and the systematically acquired corpus of knowledge based on the systematic accumulation of formal evidence, that typifies an established profession.

Why the British focus shifted

Many of the core chapters of the Seebohm report (1968) were about services. However, the Seebohm report itself was an attempt to establish the structural preconditions for most sophisticated and coordinated services at the level of the big urban authority or county, albeit an authority which was prisoner of the Bentham/Webb tradition of British public administration in its beliefs about means, and not the self-inventing institutions characteristic of the reforms of the following generation. The reason why the British reforms were able to be less service focused in general, and less SWC focused in particular, is surely that the old dynamic was effectively destroyed during the 10 years following the oil crisis. I was then complaining that many authorities had 'become caught in the web woven by their past: their goals and achievements, their investment in human and physical capital and personnel services. Meantime, ideas about the provision of services [have] moved on... It [might] be easier to encourage the development of new organisations, rather than attempt to achieve change by managerial action within the existing structure' (Davies, 1987, reprinted Davies, 1990).

Residential care fell out of favour in academic social science. Peter Townsend's classic The Last Refuge came at a time when the dislike of institutions was already growing in a wide range of areas, as Richard Titmuss had written in the Times in 1957. However, technostructure and habits of mind in the local authorities and the Ministry of Health (and later the DHSS) had ensured that they continued to develop along the SWC path on which they had started. No alternatives were being developed to cater for the gradual reduction in the number of long-stay beds in hospitals and the growing incidence of greater functional incapacity and cognitive impairment. Policy discussions lacked precision about matching the nature of SWC to differences in relevant characteristics and circumstances of individuals, and crude general general assumptions about care (Davies and Knapp, 1981). The vagueness was reflected in the concepts used, for example, 'physical' and 'mental' 'frailty'.

More important were some of the major events and currents in the policy history. Some are well known, for example the distracting expansion of intellectual horizons and the permissive increases in spending levels during the Seebohm reforms – W. J. Utting commented that the social services departments of the early 1970s were suffering from the Cinderella syndrome: a restless shift to try one bed after another. The Seebohm reforms were quickly followed by the oil crisis, stagflation and the cuts in public expenditure after Dennis Healey's visit to the IMF. Crosland's belief that the welfare state could be financed painlessly from growth was no longer tenable. Instead the academics discussed the fiscal crisis of the welfare state and how projections of public expenditure could consume unsustainable increases in the proportion of the national product (Rose and Peters, 1978). The effects for the social services included deceleration of the growth of spending, the accession of the Thatcher administration, the emergence of a new right philosophy reacting against the problems of corporatism and disliking local government, the Financial Management Initiative, leading to the establishment of the Audit Commission, and the introduction of the DHSS Social Services Inspectorate that had a 'value for money' as well as service developmental interest.

Other factors are less well known but are also important, for example pressures on unit costs of local authority provision during the high rates of growth of spending immediately after the implementation of the Seebohm proposals. These set in process a dynamic that disrupted the continuities of the first SWC-focused phase of care policy for elderly persons. From the mid-1970s onwards, authorities ceased to build old people's homes. However, there was a steep rise in their unit costs in real terms, as of unit costs throughout the social services. Amongst the reasons were that the 1970s was a period when the terms and conditions of service of public employees were greatly improved (Davies et al., 1990). Well before 1979, DHSS statistical analyses comparing averages and trends in unit costs of local authority homes with the prices charged in the private sector showed that private homes were less expensive and that the higher rate of cost increase amongst local authority homes was widening the gap. Directors of social services were anxious about the implications of some of the changes in the terms and conditions of the staff of residential facilities of the previous few years. Inside the DHSS, it was murmured that the authorities were thereby becoming increasingly vulnerable in competition with independent providers. Later, it was confirmed by academic research, and the point was taken up by the House of Commons Social Services Committee: 'a remarkable difference in unit costs for residents in local authority homes and for those supported by local authorities in homes run by other organisations' (House of Commons, 1978, p. xii).

As was predicted in the early 1980s, changes in the DHSS regulations in 1980 resulted in dramatic and sustained increases in the number of for-profit places within a few years, the rate of increase accelerating from the middle of the decade (White Paper, 1989, Figure 1). The proportion of elderly residents in private for-profit homes (authorities' own or registered independents) increased from 14 per cent in 1979 to more than 50 per cent in 1979 (Darton et al., 1987). However, it would have been naïve to infer that the price of private care would remain the same, as supply was rapidly increased in response to the increased demand and a relaxation of the rules for public payments for care. The new policy created an incentive to equalise prices upwards. The expansion brought with it a faster rise in the prices charged by private homes than in the unit costs in local authority homes so that, by 1985, costs in the one and charges in the other were on average much the same (Davies and Knapp, 1988; Darton et al., 1987; Davies, 1989). Ironically, just as academics were pouring out their cost comparisons based on old data, and the general policy community was being taught that costs of private services were on average lower than local authority costs, the costs of private provision escalated quickly. The expansion in private provision having been predicted from early in the decade, the regulations could have been amended at any time, particularly early in the decade, before doing so would have been complicated by the existence of a sector that was already large and carrying large, recently incurred commitments. Other considerations were coming into play. The concept of enabling authority, as actually enunciated in Norman Fowler's Buxton speech of 1984, was much less radical than some of the ideas circulating in the policy making community from which the Buxton speech drew.

So change was in the air. However, the effect was to expand existing forms of provision. Opportunities for new forms of provision created by changes in social security regulations during the mid-1980s were no sooner seized by suppliers than the regulations were changed again to close them off, as could most clearly be seen in the development of SWC to replace long-stay wards in psychiatric hospitals.

Therefore, what that period did was to clear the decks for implementing the post-Griffiths logic by destroying the old habits and technostructures. That made more possible the acceptance of new logics in authorities, new definitions of role and interest. In some respects, they could be seen as more likely to achieve several goals of the Seebohm age than the provision-dominated departments created in 1971.

Reform content

Some key features of the British reforms could, in the long run, be expected to lead to a contraction of SWC compared with community services.

Promoting new sources of service for flexibility and diversification, Sir Roy Griffiths argued that provision should not be the main role for authorities. Reflecting back to government the fashionable new right argument of the time, he argued that they should primarily be 'enablers' in the more radical sense meant by Nicholas Ridley than the sense in the Buxton speech, which linked with the argument of the age of Seebohm (Ridley, 1988). Diversity and new sources of services have been promoted at all levels. At the national, council and headquarters levels, for example, trade and industry policies involve the regulative framework and other policies for managing market structures and influencing its processes (Davies, 1990). At the middle management level, it is the promotion of the local development of new sources within the framework of the trade and industry policy, an activity whose unit of focus is the resource provider or the production unit: the care centre, the facility, the organisation. At the field level, care managers can use 'spot purchase' – initially the dominant arrangement – to procure help and resources, sometimes using media of exchange other than the formal payment of money to the provider, sometimes using what used to be called community development techniques rather than the market.

Initially, this feature of the policy may have favoured traditional forms of SWC more than the development of home care. It was clear from a study of policy making on the eve of the reforms that the handling of residential provision was more of a preoccupation than was the development of community services (Gostick *et al.*, in press). A major preoccupation in many authorities was whether and how far to divest themselves of their own residential provision. The government presented a double incentive to support people outside. Authorities would have to pay the total costs of those in their own provision, but only the care costs of those in independent provision. Also, the bulk of the Special Transitional Grant had to be spent on independent provision. Given the undeveloped supply of independent community service, the money could only be spent on independent residential and nursing homes. There has been a continuing rise in the number of places in residential homes provided by the independent sector (from 14,000 to 35,000 between 1989 and 1994, with further increases in the following year), but a considerable fall in the number in local authority homes since 1989 – from 107,000 to 60,000 between 1989 and 1994 – and, so the latest *Statistical Bulletin* reports, by another 8 per cent between 1994 and 1995 (Department of Health, 1995a, b). The independent providers had captured 63 per cent of the market for homes by 1995/96 (London Research Centre, 1996).

However, there is evidence that, more recently, more authorities are procuring the development of independent home care. There was a 5 per cent increase in the number of contact hours delivered by local authority home helps in England between 1992 and 1994, but a 338 per cent increase in the number of hours delivered by other providers. Over the same period, the proportion of the contact hours delivered by local authorities fell from 98 to 81 per cent (Department of Health 1995a, b). The trends continued between 1994 and 1995. All of the 8 per cent growth in home help and home care between 1994 and 1995 occurred in the independent sector, so that the proportion of contact hours it provided rose from 19 to 29 per cent (Department of Health, 1995c).

Under either of two scenarios, the long-run consequences could further erode the position of residential care. One scenario would be an increase in the independent supply of home care continuing at a high state for some years. The other would be the removal of financial incentives to channel resources into independent provision, allowing authorities to channel more of them into authority-provided home care.

A new bottom-up element of the logic

A main aim was to make the arrangements *needs-led* rather than *service-led*, with an emphasis on *user and care-giver influence and empowerment through involvement* at each stage. Again, it was assumed that making services more responsive to users' wishes would give people the choice of receiving adequate care in their own homes, and a shift of demand from SWC. One of the White Paper's priorities was to make 'the promotion of domiciliary, day and respite services to enable persons to live at home wherever sensible and feasible' (White Paper, 1989, 1.11). In the context of a perceived need to use public resources efficiently to cope with increasing numbers at risk, the switch of emphasis to providing care at home led also to the White Paper's assumption that it would be necessary to *concentrate services on those with greatest needs* (White Paper, 1989, 1.10). The concern with efficiency – in the sense of obtaining greater welfare from the public expenditure – may have reinforced the priority given to providing a choice to stay at home for more users. It was probably correct to believe that more flexible services could offer this option to many persons. It was not known how many that might be. Neither was it known how to design procedures in order to focus the home care effort on them. Also, the government and the local authorities did not at first define the expenditure limits above which they would not purchase home care, although, during the second and third year, what in effect amounted to budget limits on the value of home care packages were increasingly introduced at the local level.

Home care presents greater problems than care within a facility with highly developed individual care planning in achieving the coordination to match resources in timing and nature to individual needs. The task has been made greater by an increasing diversity of kinds of service, new specialities and the use of some agencies for filling gaps that others are unwilling to occupy. Similarly, it is complicated by the creation of an economy of care with arm's length relations between the purchaser of care on behalf of the user and at least some of the providers. Therefore, it is unsurprising that the logic required making 'assessment of need and good case management the cornerstone' device for matching resources to individual needs (White Paper, 1989, 1.8, 1.10 and 1.11).

This combination of enhanced user and care-giver influence with efficiency improvement required a continuous search to seek a better balance: a better balancing of benefits for the individual, of the interests of users and care-givers, of the interests of one client against one another, of the benefits gained from one service input compared with another. That required a new mechanism for handling the processes of interaction between users and care-givers, suppliers and those providing the finance. The documents particularly promoted budget-devolved care management in order to give those close to users – the care managers – the authority to spend, to spot purchase and to innovate in care packaging. The state papers both directly advocated these and alluded with approval to projects that were thought to embody these characteristics (White Paper, 1989, 3.3.3 and 3.3.5; Department of Health/Social Services Inspectorate, 1991). Budget devolution was treated as an issue in the inspection of care management: a desirable feature to be introduced as soon as it was practicable (Department of Health/Social Services Inspectorate, 1993, 1994a, b; Department of Health, 1995a, b). Policy thus willed the ends and promoted one of the most important means for creating processes that would make the best uses of resources at the field level.

Implications for SWC

The implications of the changes for SWC depend on the answers to two questions. First, how far have (or will) the developments of community care available to people in their own homes cause a change in the level and nature of demand for the forms of SWC available at the moment? The second question – are the preconditions sufficiently satisfied for the forms of SWC to adapt to future needs and possibilities in the best ways? – becomes more relevant the greater these changes are.

Each of the questions is extremely complex. This chapter presents only some pointers.

Post-reform changes and SWC

Authorities appeared to be slow to implement changes having a large effect on the community services during the period between the publication of the White Paper and the first phase of the reforms in 1990 (Gostick et al., in press). The general message from researchers was that such changes as were occurring were pale imitations of the idealistic models on which the reform argument was based (Hudson, 1986; Ellis, 1993; Caldock, 1994; Caldock and Nolan, 1994; Petch, 1996). Interviews with social services directors and chairs suggested that there were aspects of the values and assumptions of directors and committee chairs that threatened to inhibit them from responding to the incentives in ways which would have the most beneficial impact on users of community services (Wistow et al., 1994). Such evidence suggests that we should have to wait for some time to see a substantial impact of the reforms on community services and thus on SWC.

However, by 1993, there were signs of change. At the top of departments, there was more evidence of an ability and willingness to take advantage of the incentives even by 1993 (Wistow *et al.*, 1996). A study whose fieldwork took place in 1995 and 1996 showed which managers and workers seized on some features of the new philosophy and attempted to act on them. Discussions with three groups of persons in each of ten authorities (senior managers, middle managers and field personnel) asked each of the 138 participants to rate their priorities in their implementation of the changes. With respect to goals overall during 1992–94, most of the participants in all of the authorities claimed that the top priority had been to give users a real chance to stay at home with good care. For fieldworkers, it remains the most important goal for the period 1995–97. Their second highest priority was to enhance user empowerment. These opinions were compatible with those of new users and their principal informal care-givers. Interviewed immediately after the implementation of the first full care plan, 80 per cent of users and 88 per cent of the principal informal care-givers felt that they had had a say in the care planning. Ninety-three per cent of users and 71 per cent of care-givers stated that they thought that the care managers had understood them. Fifty-one per cent of users stated without qualification that the care managers had offered them choice, another 19 per cent stating that they were offered choice in some respects (Davies, *et al.*, 1996).

Other evidence suggests that, more recently, the reforms have indeed been changing home care services in ways which potentially make them an alternative to care in homes (Department of Health/Social Services Inspectorate, 1995; Audit Commission, 1996). That has been confirmed in a study of resources, needs and outcomes in community-based care among new users of community services and persons newly admitted to homes during 1995–96, in the authorities, the study suggesting that with the increase in the diversity of packages compared with a decade ago has come a greater responsiveness to the needs-related circumstances of users and informal care-givers (Davies *et al.*, 1995). Inspections by the Audit Commission and Social Services Inspectorate have suggested the enrichment of home care services in some authorities. Statistics for the country as a whole show a concentration of resources in bigger packages for a lower proportion of users and the rapid increase in local authority purchasing of home care from the private sector. The former is important because it suggests that services are being provided in sufficient quantity to get beyond the provision of straight-forward help with cooking, shopping, cleaning and so on. Intensive packages imply the addition of personal care tasks. One of the criticisms made during the 1980s was that the thin spreading of resources prevented this (Davies *et al.*, 1990). Now it is clear that costs of intensive packages can exceed the costs in a home, one study concluding that the costs of intensive packages are *on average* higher (London Research Centre, 1996).

The importance of the growing share of independent provision is partly that the present government protects the share of the independent sector in local expenditures, partly that the competition it brings challenges authorities' own services themselves to become more flexible, and partly that independent services are new and not as constrained by the terms and conditions and expectations of staff.

We have already described the recent but astronomic rise of the independent sector in home care: the increase in the share of a rising number of contact hours from 2 per cent in 1988 to 29 per cent in 1995. The independent sector is reported by official watchdogs to provide a more flexible service. The independent provision is being used to create more intensive service. In 1994 the proportion of recipients obtaining either more than 5 hours of contact hours per week or more than six visits per week was 15 per cent for local authority provision but 27 per cent for private provision. The proportion had increased in both sectors since 1992: from 10 per cent and 9 per cent respectively (Department of Health, 1995a). The trend continued in 1995. The same trends were evident for another indicators, such as hours per case. The proportion of cases receiving a low intensity service fell. The same growth in intensity is occurring in other community services for which it is directly measured or for which it can be inferred. For example, the proportion of meals delivered at weekends has grown (Department of Health, 1995c).

PSSRU interviews being conducted in authorities suggest that the trend is continuing: authorities are increasingly ceding a role to independent providers, so unless policy changes dramatically, the shares will rise further. The significance of that is the greater propensity to be flexible in the intensity and nature of services. The Audit Commission complain that, because most authorities continue to fund their in-house services from base budget, paying for independent provision through Standard Transitional Grant, they weaken the incentive to in-house providers to respond to care managers' requests, making the independent sector the main source of innovation (Audit Commission, 1996, para. 38).

Enrichment in the sense of 'more of the same' for some is only one aspect of the changes. It was argued that the marginal productivities of services were too low a decade ago for providing 'more of the same' to have powerful effects (Davies *et al.*, 1990). Enrichment is also a matter of increasing the flexibility of services around some ancient truths: first, the recognition of the primacy of informal care for most users (Bayley, 1973); and second the fact recognised by the Seebohm report (1968), that efficiency requires that formal and informal care be 'complementary and inextricably interwoven'. The development of special initiatives for carers, the slow adaptation of mainstream services to carers' needs, 'structures allowing for flexible purchasing', the deployment of trained staff, and 'aware, informed and confident care management' are among the factors observed to be increasing this aspect of change (Department of Health/Social Services Inspectorate, 1995).

The PSSRU study of needs resources and outcomes in 1995–96 also illustrates that (1) although differences in the needs-related circumstances of individuals dominate the selection of who receives care in homes rather than community service packages; (2) area differences of care management arrangements and process have a big effect; and therefore (3) differences between authorities now greatly affect outcomes. A decade ago, the 'before' stage of this 'before–after' study had found small area differences in who got what inputs and the effects of variations in service inputs on outcomes (Davies et al., 1990). Therefore it is likely that differences between authorities in the quality of community care have widened during the last decade. The argument is explained and the results summarised in Box 4.1.

Box 4.1

Predictors of care in residential or nursing homes or at home in 1995/96

The provision of the chance to stay at home rather than enter a residential or nursing home has been a major aim of the community care reforms. Have changes in the targeting and content of community social service packages affected who, after brokerage by the social services departments, immediately enters residential or nursing homes, and those provided with service whilst staying at home? This box reports some answers to these questions.

Data and methods

The data were from a study of people with new or greatly enhanced packages of community social care in 12 small areas in ten authorities in England and Wales during 1985 and 1986. The data are from a large study of resources, needs and outcomes in the community care of elderly people in England and Wales. The data are for the subsamples of 151 users of community services and 62 people admitted directly to residential and nursing homes for whom there was the deepest of the three levels of care manager interview. The subsample was designed to give greater probability of selection to those of greater dependency, although they covered the whole range of users. The subsample for homes entrants had a high refusal rate for those with extreme dependency. In effect, therefore, the samples are heavily weighted towards those for whom care in a home and care at home might be realistic alternatives. The data are based on face-to-face interviews by people independent of the main service agencies with users, the principal informal care-givers and personnel of the social services departments principally responsible for performing the initial tasks of case management up to the implementation of the initial post-assessment care plan.

Situations in which the pattern would be influenced by needs-based factors to an increasing degree were postulated. Figure 4.1 illustrates the argument. At one extreme, it might be possible for only needs-related circumstances to affect the probability of receiving home care or care in homes, and the kinds of needs-related circumstances affecting the probabilities would include those broader influences to which the reforms aim the patterns to respond. At the other extreme, only supply policies and constraints of the agencies might affect it. Care managers' perceptions and judgements were considered to reflect both supply and demand/need factors and were thus admitted at a second stage.

Figure 4.1

Model stage 1	Model stage 2	Model stage 3		Model stage 4
Constraints policy	Care management arrangements, divergence of perceptions and priorities between care managers and users and caregivers informal	Users' needs-related circumstances		Needs-related circumstances of informal care-givers
		Core aspects: difficulties with activities of daily living, choices support	More subtle aspects, including attitudes, wishes and	

Multivariate stepwise logic regression analysis was used to predict who obtained services. The sequence of stages was designed to allow the effects of needs-related circumstances, supply constraints and associated policy goals to be most clearly seen.

Thus there are certainly changes in community services that potentially make them an acceptable alternative to care in homes. What will be the nature of their effects on the demand for SWC in the long run?

Typically, it is likely that the degree of physical and cognitive disability of new applicants for places in SWC will continue to worsen during the next few years. However, the outcome will not be simply, or even mainly, the result of increased numbers of persons with physical dependency, cognitive impairment or even cognitive impairment with behavioural disturbances such as wandering and other security-threatening activity.

First, variations between areas in supply constraints and in the quality of particularly the care management process have an influence. The gap between good and bad practice matters. We have probably entered a period in which this gap has widened. It is to be expected that the reforms will take a long time to have their full effect anywhere. There are authorities in which the changes have been slow and not thought through clearly in terms of the new logics. These new logics are too demanding for the structures created in implementing the new policy to be borne like Raphael's Venus rising from the sea, perfect and fully formed. There are too many skills to be learned, too many artefacts to develop, too many new values to work through into practice and management. Department of Health reform documents recognised this. They argued that they would require 'a profound cultural shift', that is changes in assumptive worlds, skills and values, as well as structures and procedures. More recently, the circular *Building Partnerships for Success* asserted that 'the Government has always said that it would take about a decade for the full benefits of the community care reforms to be realised' (Departments of Health and the Environment, 1995a, b). The effect of the time lapse in the spread of good practice may be such as to leave greater demand for care in homes in some areas than in others. However, that does not necessarily follow. Authorities in the larger areas are spending the money on home care, too. They are simply not spending it in ways which can meet the needs of those most likely to enter residential care. Only some of those whose care at home will be less adequate in such areas and will, as a result, be financed by the authorities to enter homes.

Second, there is the clear importance of care-giver circumstances, particularly for those living with others. Studies of dementing elderly people suggest that user circumstances are less important than care-giver characteristics in relation to what happens; they include physical and emotional health, social support, and coping styles, the care-givers' age (Morycz, 1985; Colerick and George, 1986; Morris *et al.*, 1988; Pruchno *et al.*, 1990; Cohen *et al.*, 1993). In the short term, a combination of general but fluctuating pressures, such as the circumstances in the labour market for younger carers and the state of the housing market, will be of most influence. In the longer term, changes in household formation or the marital status distributions of the population will be great, and the factors that cause them will have large effects (Department of the Environment, 1995b; Murphy and Wang, in press). Again, the degree to which authorities are able effectively to support care-givers will matter. But the same caveat applies; it is not that authorities which do not provide the support are necessarily spending less on home care and are therefore willing to spend more on homes.

Crude changes in the roles of health services, and more subtle changes in user circumstances and other aspects of the caring capacity of the community, are of obvious importance. However, so is a factor about which less is being written: changes in SWC models themselves.

Visions for SWC

Service visions matter. They are a sheet anchor to stabilise the course when winds blow from all quarters, a compass setting and a motor to use when the weather is calm and a steady direction can be followed. At the moment, the British way of learning in SWC is too blinkered in most agencies. For example, what some directors and chairs were expressing was concerns about what was merely the danger that the British equivalent of pre-Medicaid 'mom-and-pop' homes would be forced out by price competition; they did not appear to be much concerned by the failure of radically new SWC models to appear (Wistow *et al.*, 1996). There is an over-ready acceptance of the contin-uation of virtually traditional forms of provision in much of the public and private sectors, and too much incrementalist sucking and seeing in the more innovative parts of the independent sector. The process we see has all the weakness of a purely inductive method for developing argument when the evidence is of a narrow kind from a narrow field. It is a process which insufficiently extends imaginations.

It could be otherwise. Ideas about how to match SWC to the aspira-tions and needs of users have been continuously developed in other countries, in some more than in the UK. An important way of creating a broader and clearer vision is to absorb some of the argument and experience from overseas.

'Continuum of care': a vessel being sunk by its impedimenta

If by a 'continuum of care' is meant no more than a variety of modes and packaging of care matched to the variety of needs, wishes and circumstances, the core idea is unobjectionable. However, it has come to carry intellectual baggage that distorts our vision. It has become too tied to the idea of modes and packages of care focused around levels of one needs-related circumstance only: functional disability and dependency.

One interpretation led to a model whose logic postulates distinct care modes, for example indefinite continuing care in long-stay hospital beds or nursing homes; indefinite residential care; indefinite sheltered housing with some care; and care in the home of indefinite duration complemented by respite stays elsewhere in some cases. However, each care mode could accommodate persons of only a narrow range of functional disability, perhaps a narrow range defined by more than one aspect of disability (for example, cognitive impairment with behavioral disturbance as well as physical disability), or still narrower and more specialised combinations. The same was true of the USA, as the classification by Scanlon *et al.* (1979), shown in Box 4.2, illustrates.

However, the model now has several severe limitations.

First, the concept was proposed when the systems were still at an early pre-modernist and pre-Fordist stage of development. What was then provided was a narrow range of standard options. The community care reforms were implemented partly to replace a presumption of uniformity of needs and wishes, and standardisation of response, by variety in the former, diversity in the latter, and greatly to improve the matching of resources to individual needs.

Second, studies showed that most individual care carers did not tread the path implied by the 'continuum of care' model (Hunter *et al.*, 1988).

Third, elderly people who followed such a path did so at the cost of arguably life-threatening psychological trauma, causing high rates of mortality, grief, a sense of helplessness, anger and depression during what early American reviewers of 'relocation theory' called the 'impact stage' (Yawney and Slover, 1973; Schulz and Brenner, 1977).

Fourth, the underlying reason for tying the continuum of care concepts to disability was that it was assumed that disability was the main determinant of the costs to public funds of providing acceptable care. However, one of the happy coincidences that caused reform movements around the world to be built around responding to the variety of needs is that such disabilities are only one among the influences on the costs of care. Even more importantly, they are only one among the influences on the costs of good care outcomes. The incorrect assumption is based on estimates of the average costs associated with dependency levels, but there is great variation in the costs given the small number of needs-related circumstances taken into account in the French research. There are therefore some for whom the costs

Box 4.2

Differences between the two groups

The striking features are that one-quarter even of the care-at-home care recipients had difficulties with three or more activities of daily living (ADLs), and that one-quarter of the care-in-home had difficulties with all four of the ADLs; there was a big difference between the groups in the proportion whose behaviour was disturbed due to cognitive impairment, and the median level of cognitive impairment was nearer to the threshold for severe than moderate status for the care-in-home group. The score on the burden scale may reflect the anticipated or actual reduction in burden following admission of the dependent.

Comparison of needs-related circumstances between people
(a) allocated packages of community services, and
(b) admitted to a home

(a) Number of personal care activities with which there were problems [1]

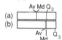

(b) Number of instrumental activities with which there were problems [2]
Discharged from hospital 33%, admitted to home 63%

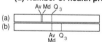

Proportions moderately impaired: at home 18%, admitted to home 32.3%
Proportions severely impaired: at home 20.5%, admitted to home 38.7%

(c) Katzman scale cognitive impairment score (0–28)
Behavioural disturbance due to cognitive impairment: at home 10%, admitted to home 44%

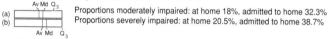

(d) Number of health problems

(e) PGC Morale Scale

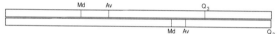

Living alone:
at home 53%, admitted to home 77%
Confiding relationship:
at home 67%, admitted to home 50%

(f) Kosberg Carer Burden Scale

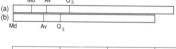

Carer–user conflict:
at home 23%, admitted to home 32%

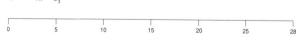

[1] (i) Washing, bathing and/or grooming; (ii) getting to the toilet; (iii) dressing and undressing; (iv) transferring to and from bed.

[2] (i) Housework and other domestic tasks; (ii) food preparation; (iii) mobility within the home; (iv) mobility outside the home.

Note: av. = average, md = medium, Q_3 = 3rd upper quartile.

in home care are much higher than costs in SWC. The converse is also true, so that one of the most important principles of budget-devolved care management is to target home care, particularly on those for whom the costs are relatively low in home care given their needs-related circumstances (Davies and Chesterman, in press).

The British seem to be learning to select for home care those for whom the quality of life as perceived by the users and care-givers themselves is likely to be good, at costs which do least damage to the capacity of the social services department to provide for the large numbers of people in great need and for whom publicly financed service would bring great benefit – whether or not, as a decision rule, it should be amended to favour home care, as suggested by the Audit Commission (1996).

Having one funding pool for the greater part of the public subsidy for community care, British social services departments have a strong incentive to balance costs against benefits in influencing decisions about the mode of care for each person. They have quickly responded to the incentive even when initially they deliberately set out to ignore it. For example, there is evidence that during the first year of the community care reforms, many authorities did not provide cost limit guidelines to care managers but that they have increasingly done so subsequently, some providing different guidelines from categories derived from the eligibility criteria (Audit Commission, 1992, 1996, para. 28). In this respect, the structures that channel practice reflect two of the principal assumptions of the reform: the need continuously to improve effectiveness and efficiency in the use of public funds, and the individuation of care. Those developing such devices for matching resources to needs in the UK came to see the issue of modal choice as requiring the individualisation of decisions unfettered by rules or expectations based on the average costs of people of different levels of dependency. In that way, the great variety of needs-related circumstances could be taken into account. Indeed, the Audit Commission have followed the Department of Health in expressing anxiety that the cost limits at which SWC becomes less expensive than home care to the authority may provide an excessive incentive to choose SWC. In other words, authorities may be giving too much weight to costs to themselves and too little to extending user choice and to the benefits for users of home care (Audit Commission, 1996).

Fifth, the quality of life remains in some important respects intransigently unsatisfactory in many forms of SWC designed around this concept of a continuum of care focused on disability. The critical literature is from several countries. The British and Americans have produced most, *The Last Refuge* (Townsend, 1962) being a true classic of policy–analytic research. The catalogue remains basically what it always was, although things have, of course, greatly improved. There is less privacy, and the strangers thrown together are not compatible. Space is more cramped and cannot be as individualised. Routines tend to become excessively rigid, around what suits staff or allows resources to be deployed at least cost, whatever the language used to justify them. Meals may be nutritious but offer little choice and are sometimes unappetising. Programmes are designed for the lowest common denominator of tastes. The forced mingling of people of different disabilities, particularly of those showing the personality and behavioural consequences of cognitive decline, causes everyday nuisances and raises anxieties. The ordinary and often unplanned activities of individual social and cultural life are relabelled 'therapies', scheduled as events, stripped of the symbolism that contributes to the satisfaction they give, and sometimes appear in extraordinary forms. The continuities of individual and social life are broken. The person is at risk of being stripped from the past, losing their sense of identity and learning to be helpless. Reactions are relabelled 'behaviours'. It can sometimes sound like a world of Orwellian 'double speak'. The exceptions that substantially avoid this are too often thought to be only for those without high levels of disability and necessarily to be costly. American evidence suggests that cognitively intact persons attach a high priority to a desire to control access to and communication with the outside world, having control over the timing and conduct of the activities of daily living (Kane *et al.*, 1990.) Is what was described for the UK after 40 years of trying to do better so different? (Willcocks *et al.*, 1987).

Finally, increasingly, those who are admitted to homes need constant health monitoring, and quick and effective access to acute health care. Even some of those which are most clearly health-related facilities – nursing homes – do not themselves provide the needed health care or give quick, coordinated access to it. The history of many in homes is of alternating acute episodes with placements in facilities assumed to provide 'long-term' care. The practice of medicine with frail elderly persons has challenges that the arrangements do not satisfy: the careful and parsimonious use of medication, the management of incontinence and its causes, the detection of illnesses presenting themselves in unusual ways, vigilance for iatrogenic problems, the consciousness of how care for the feet, teeth, vision and hearing can improve functioning, and the detection of untreated depression. Monitoring by those able quickly to observe changes is necessary for that timeliness of intervention which is so important for effectiveness among frail people. However, the arrangements lead to the neglect of these. The relationship with medicine and health care is likely to encourage not so much therapeutic lethargy as therapeutic neglect. Indeed, residents of nursing homes in the USA actually receive only moderate amounts of nursing: 70 minutes of care a day from all nursing personnel, and only 5 minutes from a registered nurse.

Some visionary glimpses: assisted living, NORCs and consumer-directed models

To illustrate some of the horizon-broadening developments in other countries, consider three American examples.

Assisted living

Some of the more progressive American states have developed a great variety of 'assisted living' arrangements – SWC which is more like care delivered in ordinary housing than homes (Mollica *et al.*, 1992; Regnier *et al.*, 1992; Kane and Wilson, 1993; Wilson, 1994).

Assisted living covers a wide variety of arrangements. However, the ideal type is conceived around designs that give those facilities which distinguish a home (a bathroom, a locking front door, a kitchenette with stove and refrigerator, and ordinary furniture), in a regime that allows as much as possible of the autonomy of life at home (allowing people to organise their space and time as they please and to take personal risks to the maximum extent) whilst providing facilities required by the more handicapped (designs accommodating wheelchairs and walking frames, two-way communications devices, congregate eating facilities – like the family restaurants attached to some Belgian homes and used like any other restaurant by those from the outside world). It also includes the flexible supply of personal and domestic care, the regular and predictable components tailor-made around the individual, perhaps increasingly delivered from the outside, perhaps provided by community home care agencies (as frequently occurs in Denmark and less frequently happens in the USA for residential and foster homes) and quasi-informal arrangements, much in the same way as might be obtained by someone living independently in the community (Hawes *et al.*, 1993; Kane *et al.*, 1993).

Oxfordshire social services department is developing models with sheltered housing on the same site as a resource centre. This could have the best of both worlds.

In the USA, assisted living has been most developed in such innovative states as Oregon. Oregon is an American state that puts a high priority on achieving positive goals through its policy-making. Its attitude to policy is proactive rather than retroactive. It strikes a new balance between regulation of inputs, and reliance on internal and external case management and the market to secure good quality; for example, it has relatively few input standards for staff or services compared with most American states. (The regulation of assisted living in a way which balances the risks against the benefits that cannot be gained without allowing them is state of the art in American policy analysis; see Wilson, 1995.) Perhaps because its citizens and politicians are interested in the welfare consequences of its policies, it has a policy for these and the services likely to produce them, as well as policy for improving access, efficiency and the restraint of growth in public spending. The policy makers are action-orientated. Its policies are thought to be efficient as well as contributing more to the quality of life of users (General Accounting Office, 1994). Other states also have seen the development of assisted living arrangements, some with state governments responding with new forms of regulation that seek to preserve rather than undermine their autonomy-enhancing features (Kane and Wilson, 1993).

The switch to an assisted living approach also encourages a change in the self-perception of the elderly person. It also changes their legal status, from that of resident to that of tenant. The implications of this are important. It entails the presumption of a high degree of autonomy and choice about day-to-day living. The professional is not assumed necessarily to know best about such matters. It is not assumed that professionals are right to restrict the risks that users take with their own lives unless they are clearly more incapable of rational decisions than the rest of us. Unlike the resident, the tenant cannot be evicted as long as certain minimal requirements are met: paying the rent or mortgage; maintenance of the property; behaving in a manner that does not cause a public nuisance. The tenant is protected by the law in the USA, as in the UK. The Fair Housing Act prohibits discrimination by disability, while health care is expected to make distinctions on the basis of disability. With this type of philosophy, programmes can push back the boundaries of the traditional residential institution, just as Oregon has done in showing how persons who elsewhere would be using nursing homes are accommodated in adult foster care and assisted living, or On Lok has done in providing clustered apartments that provide most of the cost savings in service delivery in compact areas of residential care without losing the autonomy of home life (Kane *et al.*, 1992). Assisted living can cut through the regulative barriers that reflect the assumption that there exists a distinction between residential forms of care and 'alternative' home care.

Some of the same features that define the assisted living model are also emerging in models in other countries (Pynoos and Liebig, 1995). However, it is not only the historic resonances and inappropriateness for many of nursing homes that makes assisted living seem so attractive there. Golant also contrasts the image of assisted living with the negative image of the small 'mom-and-pop' residential facilities called board and care homes in the US (Golant, 1996). Board and care homes are perceived to be amateur, socially marginal and for the poor. Golant suggests that the difficulties and dilemmas of assisted living tend to be understated and contrasts what are often the 'realities of assisted living' with 'the ideal images conveyed by its proponents'. Also, there is evidence that the small board and care home can be successful. For example, a well-conducted study of registered homes for fewer than eight residents in Baltimore and Cleveland found them to be a useful low-cost alternative in the range of provision (Morgan *et al.*, 1995).

Naturally occurring retirement communities

Having separated shelter from care, the imagination is released to develop new and resourceful forms that can transform both shelter and care by the pragmatic use of a variety of funding mechanisms. Home care can be adapted to urban ecology. The improvement of the shelter can tap housing finance streams. A striking example is the organisation of household and personal care in small neighbourhoods with high concentrations of people in need in 'naturally occurring retirement communities' (NORCs) (Hunt and Merrill, 1994a, b). By stationing home care on site, some economies in transport costs can be gained by home care. Combined with ingenuity and flexibility in tapping and using resources, innovative methods of providing support can be developed, for example the kind of improvised day care arrangements that emerged in the Kent Community Care Project in response to devolving budgets, authority and responsibility to care managers (Davies and Challis, 1986). The description of schemes of all shapes and sizes equally illustrates resourcefulness in the improvement of the housing element and in general community development.

Personal assistance services and consumer-directed models

Assisted living ideas reflect ideas generated in the care of younger disabled people. The same source is feeding ideas to what are becoming other models for elderly people in the US perhaps more than in the UK. Personal assistance is required both inside and outside the home (Kane, 1995). Medicaid personal assistance and other home care programmes funded from Medicaid waivers increasingly have targeting criteria based on measurable disability (as did the failed Clinton proposal) and the need for personal assistance, rather than on the need for specific health-related services, thereby allowing greater flexibility and client responsiveness in the selection of means and also of ends. For example, they are more compatible with the client choosing what should be the priorities between tasks. Moreover, programmes for financing personal assistance services for younger disabled people have pioneered arrangements whereby the user can manage assistants and hire and fire them, taking on those care management functions which are otherwise performed by others to the degree they want or is appropriate to their abilities (Batavia *et al.*, 1991; Sabatino and Litvak, 1992). The same ideas are being applied to elderly people (Ansello and Eustis, 1992; Doty *et al.*, 1995; Scala *et al.*, 1995). The programmes provide support to learn the necessary skills, which again greatly enhances autonomy (Litvak *et al.*, 1987; Sabatino and Litvak, 1992).

There appears to have been a surge of professional interest in *consumer-directed* programmes in the USA since 1994, one reason being the collapse of the Clinton proposals. A second reason is the realisation that much American care management has not been focused on those for whom the gains from it are greatest and has been restricted to providing inflexible responses. For many, therefore, much of the care management input has been an unnecessary additional fixed cost. Many users welcome the opportunity to undertake more tasks themselves. Thus some models are allowing variation in the care management input depending on needs and circumstances and, in so doing, are discovering the circumstances in which care management tasks can be undertaken and by whom. The British Department of Health consultation paper on direct payments is cautious, some in parliament pushing for more (Department of Health, 1996). However, it might well be that British consumer-directed models could release skilled care management for those for whom it is the best investment but for whom authorities now find it difficult to allocate the time of skilled personnel. Some American models mix degrees and kinds of consumer direction in interesting ways (Eggert, 1994).

NORCs and consumer-directed models have in common that they allow 'ageing in place' for more people than do models based on the baggage collected by the 'continuum of care' concept. Who can doubt that such models can contribute to our vision here?

Towards a new typology

Variety there must be in SWC, but since the 'continuum of care' concept has been intellectually discredited by its impedimenta, what kinds of typology would best contribute to systematic discussion of variants?

There are American analyses of congregate housing, applying elements of the reform ideas: the outcomes focus and the recognitions of the variety of needs and wishes (Golant, 1991). However, this is too narrow. A typology particularly of interest is that by Kane, who presents a classification of desired environments based on variations in people's (1) capacity for personal autonomy, (2) prognosis, and (3) likely duration of need for care. This is summarised in Box 4.3.

It leads to controversial propositions whose ethical and other implications are important to discuss.

- For those who are comatose, in vegetative states or in a very advanced stage of Alzheimer's disease, little can be done to improve the quality of life beyond giving good physical care. In such circumstances, arrangements that minimise costs and improve convenience and efficiency for staff are not at the cost of quality of life or care for the patient.
- Only those who fit the criteria for the last two rows of Box 4.3 with respect to personal care and daily living are likely to require assistance for long. For them, whether they are cognitively intact is important. Those able to use it need an environment whose physical and human resourcing allows them to direct their lives with privacy and flexibility. Those with cognitive impairment thrive best when they can exercise whatever capabilities they have for self-direction but need greater safety, cues for orientation and a simpler environment.

Box 4.3

Results

Results are summarised in the table below. Separate models are presented for those living alone and those living with others because explanatory analysis showed the pattern of influence of factors to be quite different for the two groups.

Supply/constraint and need/demand influences on the probability of receiving community services rather than admission to home

	Logistic regression coefficients			
	1	2	3	4
PERSONS LIVING ALONE				
Supply constraints and related policies				
User had needed unavailable respite care	−2.52	−1.56		
Case management arrangements				
Care manager (Cm) authority to spend		1.13		
Cm and user agreed about situation and				
help wanted		1.87	1.97	2.043
User view influenced package		2.48	2.69	2.536
User need-related circumstances				
Number of personal care activities				
with which problems			−0.306	−.0342
User male	2.06	2.22		
User tends to rely excessively on others			−1.63	−1.75
Needs of principal informal care-giver (pic)				
Plan provides support specifically for pic				1.43
Presence of pic				−1.35
Constant	1.05	−1.26	0.071	0.511
Goodness of fit				
Percentage of admissions correctly predicted				
by model	16.7	87.5	77.1	79.1
Percentage of cases for which package				
type correctly predicted by model	70.2	90.7	87.4	90.7
Significance of model c^2	0.0002	0.0000	0.0000	0.0000
PERSONS LIVING WITH OTHERS				
Supply constraints and related policies				
No variables significant				
Care management arrangements				
Cm and user agreed about situation				
and help wanted		2.36	2.77	
User view influenced package		2.36	2.73	5.56
User need-related circumstances				
User stroke victim				
Needs of principal informal care-giver			−1.91	
(Pic age)^2				0.0012
Carer balances own and user interest				4.09
Predisposing factor				
User discharged from hospital			−2.62	−3.72
Constant		.581		−1.88
Goodness of fit				
Percentage of admissions correctly predicted				
by model		0	64.3	78.6
Percentage of cases for which package type				
correctly predicted by model	No model	86.8	91.5	95.3
Significance of model c^2	significance	0.0000	0.0000	0.0000

The questions begged by such classifications consider the following:

- The handling of rehabilitation. In practice, rehabilitation has been available to only some of those requiring rehabilitation, as broadly interpreted, people from some disease categories passing along only some pathways through care systems. In the USA, both costs and results have been shown to depend on the site of post-acute treatment. However, the outcomes from lower cost settings could be improved by providing programmes in them and by delegating what other than expensive professionals could undertake after training and under supervision. In its promotion of improved rehabilitation, the Department of Health recognises the potential of social care provision. The Chief Inspector of the Social Services Inspectorate has publicised work by the National Health Service Executive and described the use of residential homes for the rehabilitation of elderly people (Laming, 1996). The NHS Executive has focused particularly on the good results from multidisciplinary stroke teams and high-quality packages for those with fractured neck of femur, explaining this exclusiveness on the lack of rigorous evaluations of other rehabilitative interventions (National Health Service Executive, 1995).
- The development of residential settings capable of coping with deteriorating functional incapacities in place, rather than by requiring a change of residence. This in turn requires both the characteristics that truly define a home and the special design and facilities required for severe disability.
- The need for a clearer distinction between (1) dependency-based classifications of residents for payment systems and classifications of facilities, and (2) the blurring of the boundaries between home care and SWC. That follows from the greater breadth in the classification of forms of shelter to accommodate changes in disability.

In many countries, there has been a trend to separate payment for (and subsidisation from public funds of) general maintenance from the payment for (and public subsidisation of) shelter and from the payment for (and public subsidisation of) household and personal care. Similarly, there has been a trend for public subsidisation to be tied to the individual rather than the form of care. One British device was the development of budget-devolved care management, in which the policy is to encourage authorities to allocate the pool of funds for payment for services to the care manager, whose care plans would therefore direct the subsidies, which would otherwise have been paid directly to providers in a lump sum. Although, in practice, local authorities are currently operating with a mix of the old and the new concept, the subsidy is sufficiently tied to the needs of the individual to allow new forms of care to emerge.

This separation out of the main cost elements for which the costs of achieving acceptable standards vary with the level of dependency of the user, from the elements that are less closely related to dependency, such as the capital and maintenance costs of design features specific to accommodating a wide range of dependency which comprise a modest proportion of the total. Again, different aspects of disability and impairment affect personal care and housing costs. This separation of payments for aspects of care therefore permits those negotiating the contracts to have a clearer perception of the relationships between costs and dependency, and to achieve outcomes from price negotiations which neither allow excessive profits nor undermine the supply of quality care in the long run.

Will the self-regulating institutions deliver?

The economic analysts of American long-term care have shown that perhaps the biggest structural obstacle to quality improvement has been the excess demand for service. That was associated with USA's attempts to keep down the rates of payment for those they financed; and also with bureaucratic styles of regulation operated in a context in which the providers were already powerful and litigious, and in which the state seemed continuously to battle against scepticism about its legitimacy as regulator. However, excess demand has not recently been a problem in most British areas, although it remains the case in some. So authorities have been able to behave in the way described for one authority by the Audit Commission: it places contracts only with providers whose provision is considered of acceptable standard and among those selecting those accepting quotes in ascending order of price until the expected demand was satisfied.

Indeed, the problem may be the opposite – the consequences of excess supply. It may be like a market for cars flooded with yesterday's models: the new car may have much more to offer, but it is just too expensive in comparison with what can be bought second hand. Most British for-profit residential and nursing homes are dated models. The loans incurred in acquiring these premises have been paid off. In contrast, an entrant wishing to provide a new form of care is also faced with these capital costs. To make the innovation worth while, the total costs of the new would have to be less than just the current operating costs of the old. This is a disincentive to providers to change the nature of their provision radically, to abandon old and constraining arrangements of the bricks and mortar and replace them with new ones. This was an important reason for the British cotton industry falling behind international competition between the two World Wars and immediately afterwards. Eventually, as profits were eroded, the manufacturers could not easily finance modernisation. Thus old providers do not have much incentive to exit, and providers of new forms of SWC have little incentive to enter the market.

Forder et al. (1996) illustrate that such barriers to exit are a common feature of the economics of markets. So are barriers to entry by new and perhaps innovative providers. The literature points to other barriers: the existing providers may rationally feel that they know the markets, have helpful reputations, be optimistic about the chances of fighting a new entrant or form of provision, or irrationally assume that what worked in the past will continue to work in the long run. It is clear that existing providers can adopt a variety of strategies to make it more difficult for others to compete against them (Dixit, 1980; Tirole, 1988; Waterson, 1988). There is no shortage of examples of the use of such strategies in SWC. The concept of the 'contestability' of the market, the possibility that new entrants may undercut prices or produce a new type of product, is key. It is only in contestable markets that the conditions for making the best use of resources are satisfied (Atkinson and Stiglitz, 1980; Baumol et al., 1982). However, there are informational and other factors preventing entry or exit when that would be in the interests of the suppliers (Nelson and Winter, 1982; Granovetter, 1985). Similarly, there is little reason to believe that suppliers' willingness and ability to learn about new models will be fast in an industry with so much of the provision made by small businessmen, often care workers applying in their own homes ideas and skills that they had acquired in old-style facilities, indeed worse, old-style health facilities.

Less attention has been paid to the effects of restricted knowledge on demand in the British argument. Perhaps it is assumed that the supplier can quickly and effectively inform users through advertising. However, that is a doubtful assumption. The context is in some ways similar to that in the market for mechanisms for risk-pooling or time-spreading for financing long-term care: the potential users are difficult to inform, tend to have beliefs and assumptions that reduce the gains they perceive the new idea to confer, and often overestimate the benefits of the alternative. The experience of the currently publicised Connecticut Partnership illustrates the great importance of consumer education rather than just the provision of information to those who seek it. There is no reason to believe that the rate of diffusion of new knowledge among the potential consumers will be fast.

Is there not the need for policy intervention to encourage and speed the systematic diffusion of knowledge and ideas about new models? There is at least a *prima facie* case to answer. Some factors affecting demand for SWC are established, as shown in Box 4.4.

Conclusions

To achieve their potential for human betterment, the changes are most often argued to require a profound cultural change. To paraphrase from a narrower perspective, what is needed is the product of innovation through competition more than simply static efficiency with current technologies (Davies *et al.*, 1990). The truth of that is becoming self-evident to an increasing number of policy makers and academics. Therefore, to move from the general logic contained in the Griffiths report (1988) to a system making it work to best effect requires not only structures and procedures, new managerial artefacts and new skills to practise the new and difficult arts implicit in the logic, but also new consumer and producer understanding of what is possible, and new visions among providers, policy makers, purchasing managers, users and users' families. There are reasons to question whether the self-inventing institutions of the market will create and disseminate the visions required without policy intervention directed at the collation of information about models and experience in other countries, and its widespread dissemination here.

Box 4.4

Implications

- Supply constraints, and priorities of authorities related to them, revealed in (1) policy and practice discussions with top and middle managers and field personnel, and (2) depth discussions of the factors influencing the care plan with people performing the core tasks of care management leading up to the initial long-term plan, did not suggest that differences between areas or cases in supply constraints were generally important, although the difficulties of providing respite care may have contributed to causing admission to homes in 4 per cent or more of cases.

- Models restricted to supply constraint variables do not successfully predict the cases admitted to homes. Those allowed to take into account care management arrangements, process variables and the needs and attitudes of users and care-givers predict 80 per cent of the cases admitted to homes.

- Features of the care management process – care managers' delegated authority to care plan within a budget, users' feelings that they had a real influence and agreement between the user and care manager about the care package – predicted the outcome well for many admitted to homes among users living alone and were significant predictors among those living with others. In part, their power as predictors might be due to the fact that most users would wish to stay at home and so would agree with a care package that would have the desired effect. However, it in part reflects the quality of the care management process leading to appropriate and flexible packages not unduly constrained by supply factors.

- For those living alone, the incapacity to perform a range of personal care activities and the degree to which the user has a personality making him or her tend to rely on others are important predictors of whether one enters a home. However, among those living with others, the ability to perform the tasks of daily living did not have a powerful effect. Having been discharged from hospital and/or having had a stroke were more powerful predictors.

- When carer-related circumstances were taken into account, the importance of the user's inability to perform personal care tasks became a less satisfactory predictor. In particular, the care manager reporting that the care package was specifically designed to provide support for the informal care-giver reduced the probability of admission to homes, an effect significant at the 5 per cent level. Among those living with others, having an older principal care-giver (perhaps a spouse or sibling) powerfully reduced the probability of admission to a home. Also, the care manager judging the principal care-giver to have a balanced approach in balancing their interests and those of the user, rather than being engulfed by the caring role, was associated with a reduction in the probability of admission to a home significant at the 5 per cent level.

- Overall, the modelling provided little support for the argument that variations in supply constraints were as important as variations in the needs/demand-related circumstances of users. However, how far authorities had delegated authority to care managers to develop care packages and differences in the quality of the care management process seemed to be of influence.

References

Ansello, E.F. and Eustis, N.N. (1992) A common stake?: investigating the emerging 'intersection' of aging and disabilities. *Generations*, **16**:49–52.
Atkinson, A. and Stiglitz, J. (1980) *Lectures in Public Economics*. London, McGraw-Hill.
Audit Commission (1992) *Exhibit 6 Community Care: Managing the Cascade of Change*. London, Audit Commission.
Audit Commission (1996) *Balancing the Care Equation: Progress with Community Care*. London, Audit Commission.
Batavia, A.I., DeJong, G., McKnew, L.B. and Bouscaren, L. (1991) Toward a national personal assistance program: the independent living model of long-term care for persons with disabilities. *Journal of Health Policy and the Law*, **16**:523–42.
Baumol, W.J., Panzar, J.C. and Willig, R.D. (1982) *Contestable Markets and the Theory of Industrial Structure*. New York, Harcourt Brace Jovanovich.
Bayley, M.J. (1973) *Mental Handicap and Community Care*. London, Routledge & Kegan Paul.
Caldock, K. (1994) The new assessment: moving towards holism or new roads to fragmentation, in Challis, D., Davies, B. and Traske, K. (eds) *Community Care: New Agendas and Challenges from the UK and Overseas*. Aldershot, Arena, pp. 133–48.
Caldock, K. and Nolan, M. (1994) Assessment and community care: are the reforms working? *Generations Review*, **4**(4): 2–4.
Challis, L. and Bartlett, H. (1987) *Old and Ill: Private Nursing Homes for Elderly People*, Research Paper 1. Mitcham, Surrey, Age Concern England.
Cohen, C., Gold, D., Shulman, K. *et al.* (1993) Factors determining the decision to institutionalise dementing individuals: a prospective study. *Gerontologist*, **33**(6):714–20.
Colerick, E.J. and George, L.K. (1986) Predictors of institutionalization among caregivers of patients with Alzheimer's Disease. *Gerontologist*, **34**: 493–8.
Darton, R., Jefferson, S., Sutcliffe, E. and Wright, K. (1987) The PSSRU/CHE Survey of Residential and Nursing Homes: The Costs and Charges of the Surveyed Homes, PSSRU Discussion Paper 563/3. Canterbury, University of Kent at Canterbury.
Davies, B.P. (1968) *Social Needs and Resources in Local Services*. London, Joseph.

Davies, B.P. (1987) Equity and efficiency in community care: supply and financing in an age of fiscal austerity. *Ageing and Society*, **7**(2):161–74.

Davies, B.P. (1989) Why must we fight the eighth deadly sin: parochialism. *Journal of Ageing and Social Policy*, **1**:217–36.

Davies, B.P. (1990) The 'trade and industry policy' metaphor and its relevance to the Griffiths Report, in Bytheway, B. and Johnson, J. (eds) *Welfare and the Ageing Experience: A Multidisciplinary Analysis.* Aldershot, Avebury, pp. 14–27.

Davies, B.P. and Challis, D.J. (1986) *Matching Resources to Needs in Community Care.* Aldershot, Gower.

Davies, B.P. and Chesterman, J. *Budget-Devolved Care Management in Two Routine Programmes: Outcomes of Two Experimental Evaluations.* Aldershot, Arena, in press.

Davies, B.P. and Knapp, M. (1981) *Old People's Homes and the Production of Welfare.* London, Routledge.

Davies, B.P. and Knapp, M. (1988) Costs and residential social care, in Sinclair, I. (ed.) *Residential Care: The Research Reviewed.* London, HMSO.

Davies, B.P., Barton, A. and McMillan, I. (1973) The silting-up of unadjustable resources and the planning of the personal social services. *Policy and Politics*, **1**(4):341–55.

Davies, B., Bebbington, A. and Charnley, H. (1990) *Resources Needs and Outcomes in Community-based Care.* Aldershot, Gower.

Davies, B.P., Warburton, R.W. and Fernandez, J. (1995) Do different case management approaches affect who gets what? Preliminary results from a comparative British study. *Care Plan*, December: 26–7.

Davies, B.P., Warburton, R.W. and Fernandez, J. with Goldstone, G., Luckham, S. and Milne, A. (1996) *Who Gets What: Service Allocations in Post-reform Community Care of Elderly People*, PSSRU Discussion Paper number 1214. Canterbury, University of Kent at Canterbury.

Department of the Environment (1995b) *Projections of Households in England to 2016.* London, HMSO.

Department of Health (1990) *Community Care in the Next Decade and Beyond: Policy Guidance.* London, HMSO.

Department of Health (1994) *Statistics of the Health and Personal Social Services in England.* London, HMSO.

Department of Health (1995a) *Local Authority Personal Social Services Statistics: Community Care: Detailed Statistics on Local Authority Personal Social Services England 1994: HMD/94.* London, HMSO.

Department of Health (1995b) *Statistics of the Health and Personal Social Services 1995, edn.* London, HMSO.

Department of Health (1995c) *Community Care Statistics 1995: Statistical Bulletin.* London, HMSO.

Department of Health (1996) *Care Management and Assessment Guide.* London, HMSO.

Departments of Health and the Environment (1995a) *Building Partnerships for Success: Community Care Development Programmes.* London, HMSO.

Department of Health/Social Services Inspectorate (1991) *Care Management and Assessment: Managers' Guide.* London, HMSO.

Department of Health/Social Services Inspectorate (1993) *Inspection of Assessment and Care Management Arrangements in Social Services Departments: Preliminary Overview Report*. London, HMSO.

Department of Health/Social Services Inspectorate (1994a) *Inspection of Assessment and Care Management Arrangements in Social Services Departments: Second Overview Report*. London, HMSO.

Department of Health/Social Services Inspectorate (1994b) *Community Care Packages for Older People*. London, HMSO.

Department of Health/Social Services Inspectorate (1995) *What Next for Carers: Findings from an SSI Project*. London, HMSO.

Dixit, A. (1980) The role of investment in entry deterrence. *Economic Journal*, **90**: 95–106.

Doty, P., Kasper, J. and Litvak, S. (1995) *Consumer-directed Models of Personal Care: Lessons from Medicaid, ASPE*. Washington, DC, Department of Health and Human Services.

Eggert, G. (1994) *Consumer-orientated Integration of Rural Health Care: A Research Proposal*. Rochester, NY, Monroe County Long Term Care Program.

Ellis, K. (1993) *Squaring the Circle: User and Carer Participation in Needs Assessment*. York, Joseph Rowntree Foundation.

Forder, J., Knapp, M. and Wistow, G (1996) Competition in the mixed economy of care. *Journal of Social Policy*, **25**(2):201–21.

General Accounting Office (1994) *Medicaid Long-term Care: Successful Efforts to Expand Home Services While Limiting Costs*, GAO/HEHS-94-167. Washington, DC, General Accounting Office.

Golant, S.M. (1991) Matching congregate housing settings with a diverse elderly population: research and theoretical considerations. *Congregate Housing for the Elderly*, 21–38.

Golant, S. (1996) Shelter and care for the elderly population: reasons for cynicism. *Gerontologist*, **36**:410–13.

Gostick, C., Davies, B.P., Lawson, R. and Walden, C. *From Vision to Reality in Community Care: Changing Direction at a Local Level 1990–1993*. Canterbury, PSSRU, University of Kent at Canterbury, in press.

Granovetter, M. (1985) Economic action and social structure: the problem of embeddedness. *American Journal of Sociology*, **91**:481–510.

Griffiths, R. (1988) *Community Care: Agenda for Action, a Report to the Secretary of State for Social Services*. London, HMSO.

Hansard (1948) House of Commons Debate, Session 1947/8, Volume 444.

Hawes, C., Wildfire, J.B. and Lux, L.J. (1993) *Regulation of Board and Care Homes: Results of a Survey in Fifty States and the District of Columbia*. Washington DC, American Association of Retired Persons.

House of Commons (1978) *Eighth Report from the Expenditure Committee, Annex v. Trends in Unit Costs for Residential Accommodation for the Elderly and the Younger Physically Handicapped 1975–76*, House of Commons Paper 600v, Session 1978. London, HMSO.

Howe, A. (1996) Community care at the margins of the acute care system, Paper presented at British Congress of Gerontology, Manchester, 3–5 July, 1996.

Hudson, H. (1986) Case management, the EPIC model: a case of not grasping the nettle, in Challis, D., Davies, B. and Traske, K. (eds) *Commu-*

nity Care: New Agendas and Challenges from the UK and Overseas. Aldershot, Arena, pp. 149–59.

Hunt, M. and Merrill, J.L. (1994a) *Naturally Occurring Retirement Communities. The Invisible Housing Alternative.* Wisconsin, University of Wisconsin at Madison, Institute of Aging.

Hunt, M.E. and Merrill, J.L. (1994b) *Rural NORC Study. A Typology of Rural Naturally Occurring Retirement Communities.* Wisconsin, University of Wisconsin at Madison.

Hunter, D., McKeganey, N. and MacPherson, I. (1988) *Care of the Elderly: Policy and Practice.* Aberdeen, Aberdeen University Press.

Kane, A. (1995) Expanding the home care concept: blurring distinctions among home care, institutional care, and other long-term care services. *The Milbank Quarterly,* **73**:161–86.

Kane, R.A. and Wilson, K.B. (1993) *Assisted Living in the United States: A New Paradigm for Residential Care of the Frail Elderly.* Washington, DC, American Association for Retired People.

Kane, R.A., Kane, R.L., Illston, L.H. *et al.* (1993) Adult foster care for the elderly in Oregon: a mainstream alternative to nursing homes? *American Journal of Public Health,* **81**:1113–20.

Kane, R.A., Freeman, I.C., Caplan, A.L. *et al.* (1990) Everyday autonomy in nursing homes. *Generations,* **14**(suppl.):69–71.

Kane, R.I., Kane, R.A., Miller, N.A. *et al.* (1992) Qualitative analysis of the Programme of All-inclusive Care of the Elderly (PACE) *Gerontologist,* **32**:771–80.

Klein, R. (1995) Self-inventing institutions: institutional design and the UK welfare state, in Goodin, R.E. (ed.) *The Theory of Institutional Design.* Cambridge, Cambridge University Press, pp. 240–54.

Laming, H. (1996) Social Services Contribution to the Rehabilitation of Older People. Letter from the Chief Inspector to directors of social services in England, CI(96)10. London, Department of Health.

Litvak, A., Zukas, H. and Heumann, J.E. (1987) *Attending to America: Personal Assistance for Independent Living.* Berkeley, CA, World Institute of Disability.

London Research Centre (1996) *Community Care Trends: The Impact of Funding on Local Authorities, January–September 1995.* London, Local Government Management Board.

Mollica, R.L., Ladd, R.C., Dietsche, S. *et al.* (1992) *Building Assisted Living for the Elderly into Public Long-term Care Policy: A Guide for the States.* Portland, ME, National Academy for State Policy, Center for Vulnerable Populations.

Morgan, L.A., Eckert, J.K. and Lyon, S.M. (1995) *Small Board-and-Care Homes: Residential Care Homes in Transition.* Baltimore, John Hopkins Press.

Morris, R.G., Morris, L.W. and Britton, P.G. (1988) Factors affecting the emotional wellbeing of the caregivers of dementia sufferers. *British Journal of Psychiatry,* **15**:147–56.

Morycz, R.K. (1985) Caregiving strain and the desire to institutionalize family members with Alzheimer's disease. *Research on Aging,* **7**:329–61.

Murphy, M.M. and Wang, D. A dynamic multi-state projection model for making marital status population projections in England and Wales, in

Dale, A. (ed.) *Using Census and Survey Data for the Analysis of Marriage and Employment Histories.* in press.

National Health Service Executive South and West and South and West Regional Health Authority (1995) *Evidence-based Purchasing: Rehabilitation of Older People.* Bristol, National Health Service Executive South and West and South and West Regional Health Authority.

Nelson, R. and Winter, S. (1982) *An Economic Theory of Evolutionary Change* Cambridge, MA, Harvard University Press.

Petch, A. (1996) New concepts, old responses: assessment and care management pilot projects in Scotland, in Phillips, J. and Penhale, B. (eds) *Reviewing Care Management for Older People,* 14–27.

Pous, J., Grand, A., Cayla, F. and Bocquet, H. (1992) L'hébergement collectif en milieu urbain, in Mire and Plan urbain *Vieillir dans la ville.* Paris, L'Harmatan, pp. 87–104.

Pruchno, R.A., Michael, E., and Potashnik, S.L. (1990) Predictors of institutionalization among victims of Alzheimer's disease victims with caregiving spouses. *Journal of Gerontology: Social Sciences,* **45**:S259–66.

Pynoos, J and Liebig, P. (eds) (1995) *Housing Frail Elders: International Policies, Perspectives and Prospects.* Baltimore, John Hopkins Press.

Regnier, V., Hamilton, J. and Yatabe, S. (1992) *Best Practices in Assisted Living: Innovations in Design, Management and Financing National Eldercare.* University of Southern California, LA, Institute on Housing and Supportive Services.

Ridley, N. (1988) *The Local Right: Enabling not Providing.* London, Centre for Policy Studies.

Rose, R and Peters, B.G. (1978) *Can Government Go Bankrupt?* New York, Basic Books.

Sabatino, C.P. and Litvak, S. (1992) Consumer–directed home care: what makes it possible. *Generations,* **16**:53–8.

Scala, M.A., Mayberry, P.S. and Kunkel, S.R. (1995) *Consumer-Directed Home Care: Client Profiles and Service Challenges.* Oxford, OH, Miami University, Scripps Gerontology Centre.

Scanlon, W., Difederico, E. and Stassen, M. (1979) *Long-Term Care: Current Experience and a Framework for Analysis.* Washington, DC, Urban Institute.

Schulz, R. and Brenner, G. (1977) Relocation of the aged: a review and theoretical analysis. *Journal of Gerontology,* **32**:322–33.

Seebohm Report (1968) *Report of the Committee on Local Authority and Allied Personal Social Services,* Cmnd 3703. London, HMSO.

Tirole, J. (1988) *The Theory of Industrial Structure.* Cambridge, MA, MIT Press.

Townsend, P. (1962) *The Last Refuge.* London, Routledge & Kegan Paul.

Waterson, M.W. (1988) *Regulation of the Firm and Natural Monopoly.* Cambridge, MA, MIT Press.

White Paper (1989) *Caring for People: Community Care in the Next Decade and Beyond,* Cmnd. 849. London, HMSO.

Wiener, J., Illston, L. and Hanley, R. (1994) *Sharing the Burden: Strategies for Public and Private Long-term Care Insurance.* Washington, DC, Brookings Institution.

Willcocks, D., Pearce, S. and Kellaher, L. (1987) *Private Lives in Public Places: A Research-based Critique of Residential Life in Local Authority Old People's Homes.* London, Tavistock.

Wilson, K.B. (1994) Assisted living: a residential model of long–term care, in Maddox, G.L., Atchley, R.C., Evans, J.G. *et al.* (eds) *The Encyclopedia of Aging*. New York, Springer, pp. 83–6.

Wilson, K.B. (1995) *Assisted Living: Reconceptualising Regulations to Meet Consumers' Needs and Preferences*. Washington, DC, American Association of Retired Persons.

Wistow, G., Knapp, M., Hardy, B. and Allen, C. (1994) *Social Care in a Mixed Economy*. Buckingham, Open University Press.

Wistow, G., Knapp, M., Hardy, B. *et al.* (1996) *Social Care Markets*. Buckingham, Open University Press.

Yawney, B.A. and Slover, D.L. (1973) Relocation of the elderly. *Social Work,* **18**:86–95.

5 THE MONASTIC TRADITION AND COMMUNITY CARE

David Brandon

This chapter continues to develop the argument that the notion of the total institution has been interpreted too narrowly and, through an historical exploration of monastic traditions, convincingly demonstrates the inadequacy of the monolithic conception of this archetypal total institution. Profesor Brandon offers instead a contrast between the reclusive culture of the Christian monastery and the highly permeable nature of the much older Buddhist tradition, with its emphasis not on retreat from the community but on the provision of care for it. The conclusion is that the marginalisation of residential forms of care in Western society can be linked to the heritage of Christian monasticism, and that the organic role of the Buddhist monastic tradition within the community provides a more creative model for residential institutions within today's community care.

This short chapter takes on a gigantic task in trying to link the development of the monastic traditions with the growth of care in the community – the care and support of those who are elderly, mentally ill and have learning difficulties over the last two and a half thousand years. There is an extremely widespread belief, perhaps even a mythology, that formal social services such as relief to the poor, homeless and sick strangers originated with monks and monasteries, particularly in the Middle Ages. The basic idea is that the early monks were embryonic social workers, teachers, nurses and doctors, and that some functions of the monasteries gradually developed into hospitals, hospices and old people's homes. For example, one powerful modern image comes from the many *Brother Cadfael* novels of Ellis Peters, now a series of TV films, which paint this mediaeval Welsh monk as a doctor, social worker and detective. This chapter looks briefly at the relevant Christian monastic tradition and then in much greater detail at both the historical and contemporary involvement of Buddhist monks in the community care field, including some direct experiences of the author.

Buddhist monasticism was very long established in northern India by the time the first Christian monks and hermits began to gather in the Scete desert, near Alexandria, in what is now Egypt, during the 3rd and 4th centuries AD (Merton, 1974). These original hermits were a movement of lay people somewhat critical of the often over-worldly life of clerics, but they also included a few important church figures such as St Antoninus. They wanted a more aesthetic and spiritual life, far away from the many distractions of the everyday priestly existence, devoting themselves more completely to the service of God in the middle of the desert. It was an important exercise in renunciation, a turning away from the everyday world:

> A certain brother went to Abbot Moses in Scete, and asked him for a good word [advice]. And the elder said to him: 'Go, sit in your cell, and your cell will teach you everything'. (Milis, 1992, pp. 44–5)

The French sociologist Moulin argued that what we call social services today was 'dispensed completely by religious people' in mediaeval times (Moulin, 1978). His view, still very popular today, is somewhat over-simplistic and contains inaccuracies. Geoffrey Chaucer illustrated the corruption of some monks and friars in his 14th-century epic poem *The Canterbury Tales*. In the view of one more recent and sardonic commentator, those religious people who lived among the poor and were also devout and compassionate were most uncommon. The majority tended to be indulgent and live a soft life (Jusserand, 1981, pp. 288–9).

The well-known monastic Rule of St Benedict, an important measuring tool, distinguished four categories of people with whom the greatest care should be taken – the sick, children, guests and the poor. However, the Rule was inspired primarily by the desire to attain eternal life in Heaven rather than by any fundamental desire essentially to serve the poor: 'Helping people out of their misery was not an issue for the monks, whose attention was focused on the after-life' (Milis, 1992, pp. 53–4). They often came from the towns and villages immediately surrounding the monastery; they knew exactly how people lived and died but were concerned primarily for their own salvation rather than with the desire to save others.

Structural relief aimed at reducing local poverty could have fundamentally undermined the whole ideal of charity, as well as dangerously
threatening important patrons amongst the wealthy land-owning
classes who financed the new buildings and much of the fabric of the
monasteries. It could have helped the peasants become wealthier and
less ignorant – seen as very spiritually undesirable and possibly leading
to dangerous social and economic imbalances.
  Monasticism in the Middle Ages was nothing if not inherently and
monumentally conservative. It was a fundamental bulwark against
change. The actual amounts of money and food distributed by many
monasteries were often minimal. To give one example, the almoner of
Christ Church, Canterbury, responsible for the care of the poor, spent
only 1.5 per cent of his budget on external poverty relief in the period
1284–1373. Other studies of the Benedictine rule show the marginality
of almsgiving for these monasteries (Rubin, 1987, p. 247). Whilst the
Cluniacs built three consecutive vast churches over two centuries
through the benevolence of rich donors, they distributed only thirty six
pounds of bread daily to the poor (Moulin, 1978, p. 291).
  Any work with the local sick and homeless people was extremely
marginal to the main functions and finances of the mediaeval monasteries, often relatively well off, to hold regular services, to pray and
contemplate, and to study and copy the biblical texts. The guests who
did receive hospitality were, for the most part, relatively wealthy trav-
ellers or pilgrims rather than the imagined poor and homeless. The
Rule defines 'guests' as important people whose arrival 'is announced'.
Concern over the sick was mostly focused on the monks who were ill
and getting elderly rather than on those from outside:

> Medical care for outsiders was not a goal of the Benedictine movement and
> in later middle ages networks of Augustinian friars or purely secular estab-
> lishments (mainly in towns) provided a more adequate health service.
> (Milis, 1992, p. 60)

  The monks held very firmly to the virtue of voluntary poverty: 'The
monks' belief in the superiority of spirituality elevated this humility to
social pride' (Milis, 1992, p. 62).
  In his famous work on asylums, Goffman defines the fundamental
characteristics of institutions as breaking the barriers between the
activities of sleeping, playing and working, ordinarily carried out in
separate locations, with separate co-participants, under different
authorities and without an overall rational plan. He divides institutions into five main types – those which care for the incapable, and
harmless; those caring for the incapable who are an unintended

threat; those designed to protect against intended dangers; those accomplishing work tasks; and finally those established as retreats from the world – 'abbeys, monasteries, convents and other cloisters' (Goffman, 1968, p. 17). Most Christian monasteries meet these various criteria splendidly. As we shall see, Buddhist monasteries meet the criteria for total institutions reasonably well, but it is difficult to see them simply as 'retreats from the world'. The monk lives in a deliberately unified system where functions of living are carried out in the same place and with the same people, but in most orders he serves the community rather than disappearing from it.

In relative historical contrast, the idea of the life of the monk, borrowed largely from the ancient Hindu traditions, arose very early in the Buddha's teachings. Whereas the Christian term 'monk' originated from the Latin *monachus*, meaning a religious hermit or solitary and only later on someone residing in a religious community or brotherhood, the equivalent Buddhist term *Bhikkhu*, usually translated as 'monk', literally means someone who receives a share of something. The Buddhist 'sharesman' had not contracted out of society; his chosen life was not just for his own private and personal benefit but a genuine form of social service to the community (Ling, 1976, p. 150).

The essential Buddhist trinity (Buddha, Dharma and Sangha) contains the concept of Sangha, meaning the community of followers and usually more specifically the monastic community. As the Buddha explained to King Agatasattu some 500 years before Christ:

> [the monk] puts away the killing of living things, holds aloof from the destruction of life. The cudgel and sword he has laid aside, and ashamed of roughness, and full of mercy, he dwells compassionate and kind to all creatures that have life. (Burtt, 1955, p. 104)

The practice of 'loving kindness' to others was basic to the life and discipline of the monk.

It was only inside the walls of the monastery that the disease of individualism could be most effectively treated, but the religious life also involved service to and the care of the various members of the community outside. Local people entered the monasteries for services, meditation classes and advice. The oriental monastic state was never the fixed lifetime undertaking that it became within Christianity, so lay people could and did become monks for a time and often de-robed without any stigma or sense of failure. There was a much less rigid distinction between the seemingly separate worlds of Sangha and laity.

Unlike the monk St Benedict, as we have seen, the Buddha accepted the practical importance of improving the existing social and economic conditions. He saw four vital elements as contributing to the happiness of lay people in this world: 'A man should be skilled and energetic in his profession; he should protect his income; have good friends; spend reasonably in relationship to income – neither too much or too little' (Rahula, 1959, pp. 81–2). It was rather more a practical vision of this world than of the next, concerned with the various complex needs of humanity.

The predominant concerns of the Buddha and his monks were with the existing and public world rather than with some mystical retreat to silence and separated spirituality. He was active in settling a number of difficult political disputes, including those over water rights. He believed that the economic welfare of his people should be a very special concern of a wise King (Rahula, 1959, p. 175). It seems clear from earliest teachings that the Buddha's ideas of the desirable state of Nirvana, as a place to find peace and freedom from suffering, were not about some distant and future goal but about the 'here and now'. The Buddha's way was essentially a healing process rather more like the contemporary therapeutic movements than what was usually understood by religions. He was more like a social psychologist and moral philosopher than the founder of a great religious movement. He asked more that people experimented and discovered for themselves than that they had faith in him and the teachings.

From the beginnings, the Buddhist monk needed a close relationship with the local lay people if he wanted to eat regularly. There were very few wealthy patrons. In many monastic orders, the monk did not plant crops or otherwise work, so could not live without the practical generosity of ordinary people, giving him food as dana. Such gifts meant that the donor could gain considerable personal merit, almost like spiritual green shield stamps. The monk also had clear responsibilities to the peasants. He instructed, exhorted and guided, trying to keep them on the path on which, hopefully, he walked himself:

> There was a widening circle from each local Buddhist sangha, a radiation of heightened morality, whose influence would, as time went by, penetrate more and more deeply into the surrounding society. (Ling, 1976, p. 171).

The Buddhist monastery in the Western world is a fairly recent phenomenon. The first monastery of any size and permanency in the UK was probably the Tibetan Samye Ling, opening in the south of Scotland in the late 1960s. In the intervening 30 years, there has been vigorous growth, more than 20 opening in diverse traditions – Theravadan, Tibetan, Zen and the Friends of the Western Buddhist Order.

I recall vividly my first experience of a Zen monastery, now nearly 25 years ago. It seemed a place of great awe and fear, of mystery and uncertainty, but it was also centrally concerned with healing and social work. The building was always cold with never enough food or drink – certainly insufficient for any real comfort. We began our long day in the middle of the night; chanting the deep sleep loudly and unmusically out of our lungs and eyes usually long before four in the morning (Brandon, 1990). We walked quietly and with dignity. We were frequently rebuked for closing doors loudly, considered one of ten thousand expressions of ego.

Our monastic day was very long and extremely disciplined. The chief weapon in the war against individuality seemed to be boredom. There was absolutely nothing to interest the ego, nothing to grasp on to – no TV or radio or films or even magazines or newspapers. Our minds desired desperately a rich and varied cabaret of hourly events and relationships. It was completely lacking. Every hour, day, week and month was much the same. We just sat for long hours cross-legged, punctuated only by the sounds of heavy breathing and the tinkling bell as the meditation leader began and ended the various interminable sessions. Each ending was accompanied with a complex ritual and a brief relief from the often intense discomfort of long hours of sitting. The knees especially became numb and very painful in alternate sessions. On getting up it was often difficult to walk.

Although we never talked to or even looked at the other monks, of both sexes, because there was usually a strict rule of silence, we developed an intimate sense of each other. We became a real community and learned to love one another. We knew when a brother or sister was struggling and suffering. I would sometimes be in floods of tears over the suffering of another monk. I got to know some people with whom I never had any conversation more closely than others, including social work colleagues, with whom I have spent thousands of hours in conversation.

There were many long sessions of *kinhin* – walking meditation, usually in the freezing dawn. We followed the meditation leader in crocodile file very close together through the spacious monastery grounds. He or she varied the pace – very fast to funereal. The considerable skill involved concentrating so completely that you never ever stepped on the heel of the person in front. It was rarely achieved, and on one very rich occasion we all fell like dominoes amid much hysterical laughter. This training was as much directed outwards as it was inwards. We were training to strengthen our concentration and awareness but also to learn how to serve our fellow sentient beings in much more skilful ways.

More difficult than the simple physical discomfort in the knees and the pains in the back were the seemingly endless tricks of mind. A voice that was rarely silent constantly told you what an idiot you were: What the Hell are you doing here anyway? What sort of a stupid place is this? You are completely wasting your time. You don't have the ability to do this stuff. I was directly face to face with my internal saboteur.

'The sentient beings are numberless, I vow to save them all.' We chanted this awesome vow many times a day. We were genuinely concerned with those outside the walls. Our salvation was entirely linked with their salvation. There was no separation. The monastery was not a castle fiercely protecting those inside from outsiders. It encouraged many visitors to attend courses, to meditate, usually very troubled people seeking some sort of solution to their sufferings. These were very ordinary people dealing with a crisis in their lives; going through the death of a child, divorce, mental illness, unemployment, a loss of meaning... , the ten thousand large and small sufferings of which human life consists – and our work was about trying to support them.

This support of the laity has a very long tradition in Buddhism. One important example of the early development of this support comes from the well-known Zen teacher Bankei, who lived in Japan during the 17th century. In his childhood, he had experienced great sorrows and difficulties and tried to kill himself by eating poisonous spiders (Waddell, 1984, p. 4). As a senior monk, he taught mostly outside the monasteries to ordinary people in their native language, whilst at that time Buddhism was mainly taught in Chinese. We have the written records of his conversations with the people who came to him.

Japanese people came with the ordinary difficulties that they might bring to a community mental health centre today – the various fears and anxieties: 'A woman asked, "I have a fear of thunder which is far out of the ordinary. Whenever I hear it, immediately I feel sick and suffer great anxiety. Please, tell me how I can somehow put an end to this fearfulness."' Bankei responded vigorously:

> When you were born you had no mind to fear things, only the unborn Buddha-mind. The illusion of fear for something is a figment of thought that was produced after you came into the world. Thunder benefits man by bringing rain into the world. It doesn't harm him. You get afraid because you contend with the thunder which is the work of that figment of thought; it doesn't come from outside yourself. When you hear the sound of thunder, trust single-mindedly in our own mind and Buddhahood. (Brandon, 1986, p. 237)

He was reminding the woman of the dangers of fragmenting attention and giving advice on how to develop greater awareness and mindfulness. Given a different language, it resembles the sort of advice a social worker or psychologist might give today: 'Fear is a social construct; don't look outside for its source, but inside.'

> During the long winter retreats many women travelled from all parts of Japan to see Bankei. Some came grieving inconsolably having lost a parent or child. He talked quietly to them. 'The sorrow of a parent who loses his child, or of a child whose parent dies, is the same throughout the world. It is a matter involving the depth of the karma binding together the relation of parent and child and making us parents and children. It is the nature of things for parents or child to grieve when death takes one from the other. Even so, for all the grief and sorrow the dead do not come back. In their ignorance, people lament continually with all their heart what cannot be undone. Was ever the return of a dead man achieved because of the zeal with which he was lamented? No.' (Brandon, 1986, p. 238)

This is an extremely tough but compassionate observation by Bankei. He is throwing a loving bucket of ice cold water over these grieving women.

The great Zen teacher next deals with a person who tells him that his advice given last year did not work.

> 'Last year when I was beset upon by confused and disordered thoughts and asked you how I could put an end to them, you told me to let the thoughts arise and cease without bothering about them. I adopted that. But later I found that it was almost impossible to do.'

Bankei despatches him firmly with, 'It's difficult because you think there's a teaching that you should let thoughts arise and cease without bothering about them. You cannot get through personal turmoil through the imposition of yet another rule, even if you think it comes from me' (Brandon, 1986, p. 239). Note the 'when I was beset upon...' as if attacked from outside by hungry and angry ghosts. Bankei deals with the 'It's your fault the advice didn't work' strategy brilliantly. Most of us, however professional and experienced, would probably fall into his cunning trap. Bankei was a sort of 17th century monk and mental health social worker, and this has remained a very vigorous tradition in modern Buddhism.

It is immensely hard to give an explanation, to put simple patterns on the painful and sometimes joyous experience of being in a monastery. Why were we there at all? Physically, the meditation posture was a straitjacket; no movement to the left or right, back or forwards. Regularly corrected by the meditation leader – moved this way and that – sometimes with great feelings of repressed rage and fury.

Our monks came like the visitors out of a sea of great troubles just as they came to Bankei. Unlike our Christian brothers and sisters, we had very little idea of what we were letting ourselves in for. Most of us were desperate; Buddhism had to be earnestly sought for in those days, not like Christianity, readily available. We were searching for both meaning and increased discipline. We had sizeable numbers of heroin addicts in the 1970s, some coming directly from detoxification units. Others had problems with addiction to alcohol. One monk had served time in prison for attempted murder. Another had been in and out of mental hospitals, diagnosed as a 'chronic schizophrenic'. Some guests came only for a few weeks, using it as a refuge before returning to whatever mess they were running away from. Others stayed for years and were eventually ordained. We were ground down in what someone called the pebble-polishing machine.

I came in to the training because my whole life seemed in ruins. It felt both empty and meaningless. I needed to find some sort of meaning and regular discipline through meditation or else I feared to kill myself. I had been suicidal and depressed for many years and could find no way out. Ironically, I worked in mental health social work and also wanted to find better and more effective methods to help others in a similar situation. If it helped me, it might help some others. I was surrounded by monks and visitors in roughly the same situation.

The monasteries were a genuine asylum for me, but it was so easy to become institutionalised. The strict and ordered regime just swept one along on a daily basis and encouraged a deep passivity. When one of the Zen monasteries partly closed down for various reasons and dozens of monks had to find work outside and live fundamentally different lives, they found it just as difficult to adjust to civvy street as any demobbed soldier or discharged long-term psychiatric patient.

On one level, the Buddhist monasteries were a kind of mental health centre for people trying to follow the Buddha's teachings on the pathway to liberation from suffering. Their income came not from begging, although they did ask for contributions from patrons, but from the running of courses and providing accommodation for the many guests and visitors. The basis of their social service was in large part the teaching of the sutras, meditation, yoga and sometimes even martial arts classes. Their thousands of students were a wide selection of seekers after truth, but many had come out of prisons and mental hospitals.

Everything in these monasteries became a device for training the monk, especially those routines which seem trivial to the outsider, including the never-ending cleaning:

> As a novice, he learns to work in the house, the temple and the garden, cleaning, cooking and pruning. A certain behaviour or deportment is expected of him. He also learns to look after the priest, to serve him and to be there for him. He learns to clean religious implements and images, often precious, to polish lacquer work, to whisk and to serve the thick ceremonial tea, to take care of the robes, both the everyday and the special ones, washing, folding, repairing and storing them. He also learns the usual Sutras [scriptures] and the chanting of them and the daily and seasonal religious observances that are held in the temple. (Schloegl, 1977, p. 31)

These diverse skills and routines were the major instruments in changing the nature of the monk's mind.

To the outsiders, monasteries of all kinds seem very mysterious and unusual places, based on strange rules such as celibacy and sanctity. They can become places of considerable projection and fantasy. To the insider, actually living there, they feel quite usual, very ordinary places. They contain the same temptations and distractions as outside. The monasteries were often not the quiet reflective and silent places imagined by the outsider. One social work friend spending a week in a monastery said she experienced more noise and grief than in any psychiatric hospital.

As well as training in Zen, I was associated for 8 years with a large Tibetan Buddhist centre that functioned both as a college and monastery. Much of that time, I taught in the centre and acted as a psychological adviser to some who lived there. What struck me most was the complete everyday ordinariness of their problems. They suffered from sexual temptation, from boredom, from longing for things and people who were not there, from despair and depression, often from an intense struggle for meaning in their lives or from the struggle with reliance on drugs and alcohol.

Most of us were in the monastery as a refuge: monks sometimes referred to it as a life-raft. Our lives outside were not working well and were sometimes going really badly. Many despaired. We felt a failure at our jobs, at relationships, as fathers, mothers, husbands and wives, that we were not genuinely worthwhile human beings but synthetic fakes. We felt a surging of deep suffering and each in various ways sought for some genuine peace of mind. Some, like me, had reached the depths and tried to kill ourselves. Others had been in various institutions. Some were on the run, unable to live with any comfort with ourselves or any others.

The great parable of the mustard seed captures the essence of the involvement of Buddhist monks in the ordinary world of everyday suffering. Gotami came from a poverty-stricken home to marry her richer husband. Until she gave birth to a son, she was treated with great disrespect by his family. But when the son was old enough to play, he died suddenly.

> She was sorrowful beyond any words. She wandered around with her dead son on her hip crying, 'Give me medicine for my son'. A wise man living locally took pity on her and sent her to the Lord Buddha, who was staying in a nearby monastery. She took her dead son with her and begged the Buddha, 'Give me medicine for my son'.
>
> The Great Teacher saw how she was and the vast extent of her deep grief. 'You did well to come here Gotami. Go and enter the nearby city and from whatever house that nobody has died, fetch tiny grains of mustard seed'. She was joyful and at the first house visited asked: 'Give me mustard seed to take to the Great Lord'. When they brought the seed she asked if anyone had died and of course at every house someone had died. In every case, she had to refuse the seed and so at the end of the day, very tired, after visiting many houses, her bowl was quite empty.
>
> Completely overcome with emotion, she went outside the city, carried her son to the burning-ground, and holding him her arms, said: 'Dear little son, I thought that you alone had been overtaken by this thing which men call death. But you are not the only one death has overtaken. This is a law common to all mankind'. She cast the body of the child in to the burning-ground and then went to ask the Buddha for refuge – to follow him. (Burtt, 1955, pp. 43–6.

The role of the Buddhist monk lies within this earthly world, walking firmly on the soil, not retreating to some mystical and airy existence. He tries to heal, to make whole by bringing together the fragments of the other. The Buddha saw clearly the immense sorrow of Gotami and recognised her capacity for growth, even for enlightenment. He sets her a test to show her that she is not separate in her grief but joined to all others. She sees this essential unity and uses it to accept the death of her small son and to develop compassion in order to serve herself and others more effectively.

In this chapter, we have looked at some popular myths about monasteries in the Middle Ages and questioned how far they were really involved in social service to the peasants living close by and from among whose families they were so often recruited. Were they mediaeval social workers and healers? We studied the development of Buddhist monasteries and their monks or Bhikkhus, beginning two and half thousand years ago in the teachings of the Buddha. These monasteries are certainly total institutions in the Goffman sense but were and are still extremely diffusive, the monks coming out to beg for alms as well as serving the community through courses, medical facilities, and even in one case, through a bakery making bread for homeless people. They were never a retreat from the world in the Christian sense. These religious institutions and the surrounding communities are interdependent. We concluded with some personal reflections on being a monk and the famous parable of the mustard seed.

References

Brandon, D. (1986) Bankei – seventeenth century – social worker, in Claxton, G. (ed.) *Beyond Therapy*. London, Wisdom, p. 237.

Brandon, D. (1990) *Zen in the Art of Helping*. Harmondsworth, Arkana.

Burtt, E.A. (ed.) (1955) *The Teachings of the Compassionate Buddha*. New York, Mentor.

Goffman, E. (1968) *Asylums – Essays on the Social Situation of Mental Patients and Other Inmates*. New York, Anchor Books.

Jusserand, J.J. (1981) *English Wayfaring Life in the Middle Ages*, 8th edn. London, Fisher Unwin.

Ling, T. (1976) *The Buddha*. Harmondsworth, Penguin.

Merton, T. (1974) *The Wisdom of the Desert*. London, Sheldon Press.

Milis, L.J.R. (1992) *Angelic Monks and Earthly Men*. Woodbridge, Boydell.

Moulin, L. (1978) *La Vie Quotidienne des Religieux au Moyen Age, Xe-XVe siècle*. Paris.

Rahula, W. (1959) *What the Buddha Taught*. London, Gordon Fraser.

Rubin, M. (1987) *Charity and Community in Medieval Cambridge*. (Cambridge Studies in Medieval Life and Thought, Fourth Series), Cambridge.

Schloegl, I. (1977) *The Zen Way*. London, Sheldon Press.

Waddell, N. (ed.) (1984) (trans.) *The Unborn – The Life and Teaching of Zen Master Bankei: 1622–1693*. San Francisco, North Point Press.

6 RESPITE CARE IN HOMES AND HOSPITALS

Jo Moriarty and Enid Levin

This chapter and the two that follow examine specific functions of residential care locating them within the system of formal and informal institutions that contribute to the production of welfare in society. Continuing the theme of the previous two chapters of the potential permeability of residential and community-based care, Jo Moriarty and Enid Levin emphasise the interdependence of both forms of care and informal caring networks. They suggest that the neglect of this systemic view has led to a limited understanding of the potential, specific role of this form of provision. As in previous chapters, the conclusion that emerges from analysis of their own research and that of others in the UK and abroad is that the continued development of this type of residential care is essential to the maintenance of caring communities.

Definitions of what constitutes a respite care service vary. Nevertheless, they customarily share the primary aim of enabling those looking after a member of their family or a friend to take a break from caring. As such, they can be provided across several settings, both within and outside the home. In this chapter, we propose to concentrate upon a specific form of respite care: that which is provided at least overnight but can be extended upwards to a period of several weeks in all forms of institutional setting, by which we mean residential and nursing homes and hospital wards. The content will be mainly drawn from the literature on older people. We shall make particular reference to the Department of Health-funded studies of people with Alzheimer's disease or a related disorder and their carers, which we ourselves have completed

(Levin *et al.*, 1989, 1994). Our aim is to locate the discussion about the nature and purpose of respite care in homes and hospitals firmly within the context of its relationship with other community and residential provision. We hope that this will lend support to our viewpoint that such respite care has a distinct identity differentiating it from other arrangements designed to help people with disabilities and their families. Neglect of these issues contributes to a lack of specificity about its purpose. It also results in a tendency to underestimate the role it plays in bridging the gap between those services that are provided in the community and those that are not.

Terminology

The expression 'respite care' has itself increasingly come in for criticism. For some, the expanding variety of services each with a range of aims means that the word has outlived its usefulness. For others, the phrase is implicitly distasteful, implying that the user is a burden from whom the carer must be relieved (Stalker, 1996). This is why increasing preference is given to the terms 'short stays' or 'short-term breaks' (Social Services Inspectorate, 1993). Whilst acknowledging the validity of this viewpoint, we shall retain the use of the word 'respite' whenever we refer to care provided for any period greater than 24 hours whose chief purpose has been to provide a break for the carer. This is for two reasons. First, 'respite' seems to have a wider currency, certainly outside the UK. Second, 'short-term care' has often been used to cover a wide range of admissions to homes and hospitals. As we hope to show, it is the failure to separate out factors relating specifically to respite from wider questions about the nature of care in homes and hospitals that has served to muddy the waters of our ability to evaluate its effectiveness.

The development of respite care in homes and hospitals

The origins of respite care in institutions can be traced back to the early days of the NHS. In 1948 Sheldon suggested the use of short-stay hostels to support the carers of disabled older people. Almost 10 years later, De Largy (1957) argued that because many admissions to acute geriatric care occurred when carers were no longer able to carry on, the solution was to provide older people and their families with periodic planned breaks. Allen's (1983) seminal study of local authority residential homes commented that, in the past, many inner city boroughs ran seaside holiday homes for the use of 'a rather younger, fitter group of elderly people than those entering residential care'. This practice was being taken forward, she reported, with the establishment of units that were now 'offer[ing] the type of care needed by the frail elderly [for a short term]'. It has been suggested that this pattern of service development can also be found in the field of children with learning difficulties (Oswin, 1984).

Provision of these types of break as a proportion of all stays in residential care, particularly in homes run by local authorities, rose steadily throughout the 1970s and 80s. At the same time, we can also see the influence of the wider movement that is the predominant theme of other chapters in this book. Based on an idea that had originally developed in Scandinavia, the first family-based short-term care schemes started in the UK in the mid-1970s. They involved arrangements for the recruitment and payment of individuals to provide breaks in the setting of their own home for adults and children with disabilities (Robinson, 1991). She has since reported that the most recent figures suggest that there are now over 250 of these schemes in Great Britain, providing places for approximately 10,000 children (Robinson, 1996). Despite this expansion, it would be hard to argue convincingly that family-based respite care has become part of mainstream provision. The majority of schemes are directed at helping children, yet even so Robinson quotes evidence to suggest that places are heavily over-subscribed. There are also other options, such as holidays provided by the Winged Fellowship Trust or finding a hotel able to provide for guests needing personal or nursing care. However, the level of demand that can be met in this way is likewise limited. This means that many people with disabilities and their families still look to residential and nursing homes and hospitals when they are seeking to arrange breaks for longer periods.

Respite care: part of a continuum

This situation raises a fundamental question about the nature of respite care in homes and hospitals. As we have seen, its development was underpinned by an assumption that it would help to sustain caring relationships, thereby enabling people with disabilities to continue to remain at home. As such, community living was to be achieved through the provision of care in an institutional setting. This typifies the difficulties inherent in defining what is a community service and what is an institutional one. Organisations such as the Carers' National Association and the Alzheimer's Disease Society regularly point out that the majority of long-term care continues to be provided by so-called informal carers to people living in their own homes. As Townsend pointed out 34 years ago:

> This question [of the stage at which people should be admitted to institutions] has become increasingly difficult to answer in recent years because we have begun to realize that there is no natural division of the elderly into a home and an institutional population. (Townsend, 1963, p. 222)

We can see that, from the start, developments in respite care in homes and hospitals were designed for groups such as older people with multiple disabilities or adults and children with learning disabilities. These were, of course, precisely those people who made up a large proportion of residents in the old long-stay hospitals. Later parts of this chapter will develop these points more fully. For now, we shall simply raise the question that, if the users of a service are primarily those who can be identified as likely to need sustained and intensive forms of support to remain living at home, is it not likely that the underlying purpose of respite care is not solely preventative but also to delay the point at which admissions to any form of residential care are likely to occur?

What should be the analytical framework for evaluating respite care?

We would suggest that there are three factors that explain why many of the existing studies of respite care in homes and hospitals are unsatisfactory, both in their scope and in the assumptions upon which they have been based. This means that their usefulness can only be limited. First, we have already mentioned the problem of a lack of specificity about its purpose. This criticism is by no means new. Brodaty and Gresham have suggested that:

> Lack of specificity in the choice of respite care may obscure demonstration of any benefit... As in clinical medicine, objectives need to be clarified and comprehensively discussed before prescriptions are written. (Brodaty and Gresham, 1992, p. 361)

Besides, if we see respite care in homes and hospitals as nothing more than a means of giving carers a break, this minimises the potential for identifying other possible benefits, such as the:

> opportunity to attend to other needs of carers, such as information, skills training and emotional support... . Furthermore, there is a need to provide an experience which is meaningful for the... user. (Nolan and Grant, 1992, p. 229)

The second point relates to the paucity of studies with an evaluative design. This is a problem that has been regularly identified in reviews of the literature (Twigg *et al.*, 1990; Twigg, 1992; Twigg and Atkin, 1994). Whilst there is no doubt that the descriptive account of a single service had a valuable role to play in building up the exchange of information and ideas and is likely to have a continued relevance at the local level, it lacks generalisability. Its inherent limitations are demonstrated by the increasing interest in developing new methodologies that incorporate the views of service users at all stages of a study design (see, for example, Darnell *et al.*, 1996) or the work on the feasibility of incorporating a greater focus on outcomes into routine evaluations of service provision or audit (Ramsay *et al.*, 1995; Qureshi and Nocon, 1996).

Finally, few studies have analysed the impact of respite care in homes and hospitals against the backdrop of the full range of service provision. Where this has been possible, a clearer picture of differences, similarities and service preferences has emerged (Levin *et al.*, 1989, 1994; Challis *et al.*, 1995).

Differences between types of respite care

What is our evidence for suggesting that this should be the case? We believe that respite care in homes and hospitals can be contrasted with other forms of respite provision, both qualitatively in terms of how it is perceived by different carers and users and quantitatively in terms of the way in which service users can be demonstrated to differ from non-service users.

From the perspective of carers, respite care in homes and hospitals offers the opportunity for a much longer break than that traditionally afforded by day care or sitting services and other home-based schemes. Yet they may spend its duration experiencing several potentially conflicting emotions: guilt and anxiety that the person cared for may not like the venue, a sense of loss or purpose whilst he or she is away, and pleasure or freedom that their time is their own (Twigg *et al.*, 1990;

Twigg, 1992). As one daughter interviewed in our study of resident carers of people with Alzheimer's disease or a related disorder explained:

> I always feel guilty when she goes. Then when she's gone, I feel free. (Levin *et al.*, 1994, p. 110)

We also found that it was possible to predict which carers had tried respite care in homes and hospitals. Daughters were significantly more likely to use the service than were spouses. In contrast, only those spouses who were experiencing the greatest difficulties in terms of their psychological health, as measured by the General Health Questionnaire (GHQ-28) (Goldberg and Williams, 1988) and the degree of restriction that they reported, were likely to be using this form of care. Among non-users, offers of the service were not related to kinship tie, so we did not believe that this finding was explained by statutory sources focusing their attentions on daughters rather than spouses.

The influence of kinship tie on the use of respite care in homes and hospitals may be an artefact of research restricted to older people. Among their carers, spouses and daughters predominate (Qureshi and Walker, 1989; Arber and Ginn, 1991). Additionally, other kin relationships are also likely to be involved. This differs from adults and children with a learning disability where the overwhelming majority of carers are likely to be parents.

Clear differences emerged when those whose service packages included respite care in homes and hospitals were compared with those who did not. Our analyses suggested that it was a service targetted at those who were experiencing the greatest difficulties with their role as carers and/or who were caring for people in the more advanced stages of Alzheimer's disease. On average, use of the service began about 6 months later than the equivalent figures for day care and sitting services. The number of carers who used respite care in homes and hospitals in isolation from day care or sitting services was in single figures, suggesting that it was offered when the regular weekly input of day care and/or sitting proved insufficient. Thus, it was a service designed to help those who were *already* at risk of entry into some form of residential care.

In this way, we identified evidence of the role it could play as a transitional service, bridging the gap between community and services and residential care settings. The suggestion that it may be used to delay or ration admissions to residential or nursing care is consistent with the findings from an earlier study (Levin *et al.*, 1989) and with reviews of the literature on respite care in homes and hospitals for people with dementia (Archibald, 1996).

As we have already commented, residential respite was, in the past, overwhelmingly provided within the statutory sector in NHS wards and local authority homes. Now, the advent of welfare pluralism has created a less monolithic picture. So does it really matter in which sector care is provided? Our answer to this would be 'yes'. When we grouped the older people with dementia into those who received respite care in the NHS, those who used residential and nursing homes and those using family-based care, the differences between the groups were apparent. At one end were the family-based respite care users, less cognitively impaired, continent and not displaying any of the behavioural problems that can occur in Alzheimer's disease or related disorders. At the other end were those who received respite care in NHS continuing care wards who, on the basis of the measures that we used, were very much more likely to be severely affected by their illness.

Our final piece of evidence to support the concept of respite care in homes and hospitals as a phased service with a staged introduction stems from our comparison of service utilisation at Time One, when the carers were first interviewed, and Time Two, when the second interviews took place, which was around a year later. On the whole, despite the progressive nature of Alzheimer's disease, service provision for those in the sample had changed very little. The one exception was the use of respite care in homes and hospitals. Many carers who stated at Time One that they neither used the service, nor indeed wished to, had begun to do so by Time Two.

Why should this have happened? One interpretation is that caring for a person with Alzheimer's disease or a related disorder over a number of years may ultimately contribute to a 'wear and tear effect' upon carers' mental health (Schulz and Williamson, 1991). The effect of this may be to break down any natural resistance that exists against placing the person for whom they care in a home or hospital, albeit temporarily.

User and carer views of respite care in homes and hospitals

Who benefits?

In our study, nearly all the carers identified positive effects from sitting services and day care on the older person, such as increased stimulation and company. In so far as respite care in homes and hospitals was concerned, many carers went to lengths to explain that they saw it as a service primarily designed to help *them*. One wife explained that her husband:

didn't want to go but he accepted it for my sake.

Others reported that they would tell the older person that he or she was going away for a check-up or on holiday.

The nature of our sample meant that, although they were asked, few of the older people were able to remember details of their stay or how they had found it. Information on how such stays are experienced by older people themselves *was* obtained by Nolan and Grant (1992). Part of their wide-ranging study included collecting the perspectives of staff, carers and older people in a geriatric hospital. From the information obtained in interviews with a group of 30 older people, the authors categorised the participants into three groups. The largest group (n = 17) consisted of those who tolerated their stay on the basis that it was to be for a limited period of time. The seven people for whom it had been a positive experience were classified as beneficiaries. For the remaining six, the experience had been totally negative.

The views of adults with a learning disability who have experienced short stays in homes and hospitals have been recounted by Darnell *et al.* (1996). For them, what was disappointing was not ensuring that 'taken-for-granted' aspects of their everyday lives could be continued whilst in respite care. These included the loss of privacy because there were no individual rooms, inflexible routines (bedtime at 7.00 p.m.), lack of activities and the failure to engage with individuals to such an extent that staff did not even know what type of food they preferred.

Twigg and Atkin (1994) have commented that the concept of respite care, as opposed to befriending schemes, is almost entirely absent for people with mental health problems. It has been suggested that a guest house in Scotland providing people with mental health problems with stays of up to 3 weeks is probably unique (Petch, 1996). Those who used the service were overwhelmingly positive in their views. Set against this picture must be the limitation that so few people would be able to benefit from such an opportunity.

Do people deteriorate as a result of respite care in homes and hospitals?

Whenever the topic of respite care in homes and hospitals is mentioned, two problems emerge with an almost inevitable regularity: how to deal with lost possessions, and whether the stay away has resulted in the person being cared for deteriorating. On an individual level, just one account of somebody returning home in a worse state than when they left is devastating. What does it also say about this system of care as a whole?

Our sample of 287 carers (Levin *et al.*, 1994) included 149 who had tried respite care in a home or hospital, 12 who had used residential and family-based respite and six who had used family-based respite only. They were all asked about their experience of the service, and in particular their last break, in great detail. The overwhelming majority reported that they believed that the stay had made no difference, although many attributed this to the severity with which the person they cared was affected by Alzheimer's disease. Eleven per cent reported a deterioration, and a third felt that the person had benefited. The most frequently reported changes were increased disorientation and finding it hard to revert to the 'home' routine. These problems were almost always believed to be temporary.

In contrast to our picture of a 'neutral' effect of respite, a Canadian study of older people randomly assigned to respite care in nursing homes or on a waiting list found that, regardless of whether or not the person had dementia, the respite group *improved* in terms of their cognitive and physical functioning when compared with those on the waiting list (Burdz *et al.*, 1988).

Service quality and alternatives to respite care

So far then, our picture of respite care in homes and hospitals suggests that it is a way of offering those carers who are experiencing stress a better chance of a break which is generally appreciated by them. While the claim that long-term damage results is unproven, why then should its reputation often seem to be that of the poor relation when compared with other forms of service?

It would seem to us that there are two reasons. The first is that more work is needed on disentangling causes of dissatisfaction in order that they can be remedied. All studies of respite care in homes and hospitals have produced a number of criticisms (Levin *et al.*, 1989, 1994; Nolan and Grant, 1992; Robinson, 1996). Problems include a poor physical environment, neglecting aspects of personal care (such as not helping the person to change his or her clothes) and not ensuring that his or her possessions are safe. Where people have problems in making their views known, additional obstacles are caused by, in the words of Nolan and Grant (1992), ignoring the 'carer's expert knowledge' on, for example, preferences and personality traits. In terms of the way in which breaks are provided, lengths of stay can be inflexible (the '2 weeks in, 6 weeks out' pattern), and carers and those for whom they care are often inadequately prepared prior to the stay. This last point is where family-based schemes constantly seem to score over residential respite venues. Thorough preparatory work takes place on matching up families with each other and establishing contact before the stay begins (Levin *et al.*, 1994; Robinson, 1996).

Some of the issues outlined above relate directly to respite stays. As an example, some people would prefer a long weekend to stays of a fortnight. Equally, it should not be impossible to arrange for the person who is to spend time away from home to visit places in advance and choose where he or she will go. However, some items on the list seem to say more about the overall quality of care in the home or hospital than about respite care *per se*. For example, residential and nursing homes now deal with people with higher levels of need than in the past. It may be that staff training and support has not kept pace with these changes (Baillon *et al.*, 1996). In addition, Robertson *et al.*'s (1995) study of continuing care wards suggested that a strong relationship exists between job satisfaction and quality of care. It may be that to focus attention upon improving standards in these areas could have a positive effect upon improving the experience of those admitted for a respite stay, as well as for permanent residents.

The second difficulty is that deficiencies in respite care in homes and hospitals may actually reflect a failure to develop adequate community-based alternatives. When respite care began, most capital resources in the NHS and local authorities were buildings-based; there was a relatively ready supply of beds that could designated as 'respite'. Failure to meet the demand for suitable community alternatives for people with disabilities and their families meant that unsuitable offers of respite were made. This left people with two options. The first was to take whatever was available. Robinson and Stalker (1993) reported that where children made multiple use of residential care 'this was usually to meet parents' needs for a higher level of support than was available in any one setting'. The second was to take nothing. Qureshi's (1992) study of parents of young adults with learning and behaviour difficulties in the north west of England identified instances in which the care that was offered was on such unsuitable terms that carers refused it – in some districts, all that was available was a bed in the regional special hospital. Indeed, the total service use by those in the sample:

> emphasizes the relative insignificance of the whole of the formal sector in comparison with the parents of these young adults. (Qureshi, 1992, p. 109)

This brings us to the final issue in this section; the potential for conflict between someone's right to live as an autonomous human being and the need to take account of the interests of that person on whom they may rely for a large proportion of help on a daily basis. Twigg and Atkin (1995) use the term 'moral status' to encapsulate the ways in which different medical conditions can affect the balance of interests between the carer and the cared-for person. They argue that the perceived moral status of the cared-for person in terms of the interaction between the two elements of mental competence and achieved adulthood will always have consequences for the negotiation of services, affecting the attitude of carers and service providers. Because of its connotations of being 'sent away', respite care in homes and hospitals is a form of care in which the tensions between the two are very strongly apparent.

Use of respite care and placement in residential settings

An unintended consequence of the early enthusiasm for having identified a method of supporting carers *and* avoiding admissions to residential care was the failure to identify suitable means by which to measure whether or not these aims were being achieved. This meant that when studies of carers of people with Alzheimer's disease or a related disorder (Scharlach and Frenzel, 1986; Levin *et al.*, 1989; Melzer, 1990) and of carers of learning disabled adults with severely challenging behaviour (Qureshi, 1993) suggested that the use of respite care in homes and hospitals resulted in more *frequent* placements in residential settings, the results were sometimes viewed as being counterintuitive.

Such findings must always be interpreted by taking account of how the characteristics of those using the service differ from those who do not. It is also likely that the experience of respite care in homes and hospitals may help to dismantle the barriers towards permanent placement, that it is, in effect, a dry run. However, is it respite care in homes and hospitals that increases the rate of progression to some form of residential care, or is its introduction simply a recognition of the probable next step?

Kosloski and Montgomery (1995) argue that the process of evaluation is constantly unfolding. In the early stages, it may only be possible to identify particular phenomena. Later work may explain the underlying fundamental processes and highlight the need to reconsider the first set of findings. For example, in 1989 Montgomery and Borgatta reported on their study in Seattle. Over 500 older people and their families had been randomly assigned to one of five groups eligible for respite and/or educational programmes or to a control group of non-service users. The results suggested that spouses, but not adult children, who participated in the programmes were more likely to place their partner in a nursing home (Montgomery and Borgatta, 1989). Later re-analyses suggested that the probability of nursing home placement *decreased* in line with an increase in the use of respite (Kosloski and Montgomery, 1995). Nevertheless, positive as this finding is, it must be treated with a certain amount of circumspection; an increase of $100-worth of respite care produced a 1 week delay in institutionalisation!

In some ways, our own experience was similar (Levin *et al.*, 1994). One of the reasons for the second study was to shed further light on the finding that people using respite care in homes and hospitals at Time One were more likely to be living there permanently by Time Two (Levin *et al.*, 1989). The first univariate analyses also suggested a positive relationship between the receipt of respite care in homes and hospitals at Time One and an outcome of admission to some form of residential care by Time Two. However, the second study had larger numbers than the original, and this relationship disappeared when controlled for in a multivariate analysis. The variance explained by the final logistic regression model was 53 per cent, with an overall prediction rate of 89 per cent. In ascending order of importance was the age of the older person, the carer's GHQ score, the older person's dependency, as measured by their scores on the Behaviour Rating Scale and Information and Orientation Questions from the Clifton Assessment Procedures for the Elderly (CAPE) (Pattie and Gilleard, 1979), and whether or not the carer would have accepted an offer of residential care at first interview. Furthermore, we also identified a group of older people receiving respite care in homes and hospitals who were very unlikely to have entered some form of residential care by Time Two. Interestingly, in the light of Kosloski and Montgomery's findings, these were the group who had been using the service for over a year at the time of the first interviews.

From this, we would argue that it is likely that users of respite care in homes and hospitals can be divided into subgroups. There are those for whom it is a way of helping them to stay at home. At the same time, there are others who are offered temporary stays as a holding measure while the process of arranging a more permanent place is made. It is important, therefore, not to make global assumptions about the service.

Discussion

The history of respite care in homes and hospitals mirrors many of the wider developments in the field of health and social care. Early enthusiasm for providing short-term admissions to homes and hospitals stemmed from an acknowledgement that there were as many people with severe disabilities living in the community as there were in institutions. In terms of Twigg's model (1989) of how agencies conceptualise their relationship with carers, early concerns were with the maintenance of carers as a resource; providing a break would help them to continue. As the strength of the disability movement grew, the idea that it was acceptable to ask someone to move out of his or her home for a fortnight every 6 weeks or so was challenged. New ideas of good practice evolved in residential homes. Was it right that permanent residents should be expected to live alongside a constantly changing group of people?

It was an essentially public form of provision, predominantly provided in local authority homes and hospital wards. Those who used the independent sector generally made their own private arrangements and did not involve statutory agencies. As with all community services, availability was patchy and was often only the result of a great deal of local lobbying. Although new forms of home-based care were developing, availability was easily outstripped by demand.

The legitimisation of respite in the forefront of service aims came with the publication of *Caring for People* in 1989. The first of its key objectives was:

> to promote the development of domiciliary, day and respite services to enable people to live in their own homes whenever feasible and sensible.

To what extent do families' everyday experiences suggest that this has been achieved since the final implementation of the National Health Service and Community Care Act 1990? It is probably too early to see whether the closure of local authority homes and hospital wards has led to a large-scale shift to move community-based schemes such as sitting and family-based care into the mainstream. Henwood *et al.*, (1996) report that whilst some of the focus groups with whom they have been working related some progress, but:

> with the exception of a few individual examples, hard evidence of service improvement was thin and the belief in improvement was not always grounded in firm data. (p. 44)

Has there then been a reduction in this form of care? Some would argue that the emphasis in the guidance document on NHS responsibilities for meeting continuing health care needs (HSG(95)8/ LAC(95)5, 1995) on the need to make arrangements to fund respite health care is a recognition that a balance needed to be redressed. In view of the complex health and social care needs of those who were likely to have used respite care in homes and hospitals in the past, it is clearly important that their needs continue to be recognised.

The literature on respite care in homes and hospitals is limited, often restricted to small-scale local studies. Few projects have adopted an evaluative design. In particular, the lack of studies across different groups of users means that we know very little about whether a form of service provision for one client group is transferable to others. Nevertheless, existing research does have some messages to help identify whether respite care in homes and hospitals should have a role in the future.

First, comparisons of the needs of users and non-users suggest that it is not a service that can easily be substituted by less intensive forms of provision. Second, carers using the service are also likely to differ from those who do not. As with most service, universal suitability is unlikely. It may not be in line with the wishes of, say, partners who want to remain together, but it can be appropriate for those who are experiencing stresses and difficulties that cannot be relieved by a shorter period of respite. This brings us to our third point. It is unlikely to be used in isolation from any other community service, so cannot be considered in isolation. Fourth, there is a need to try to ensure that it is a positive experience for those who are cared for. Fifth, there is a need to separate problems that are inherently related to respite care (unfamiliar environment, loss of usual routines and so on) from those which reflect wider problems in the service (staffing levels and physical environment). Finally, 'respite' care in homes and hospitals can be provided for a variety of reasons. If we do not acknowledge the multiplicity of service aims, we shall continue to have problems in measuring whether these objectives are met.

References

Allen, I. (1983) *Short Stay Residential Care for the Elderly*. London, Policy Studies Institute.

Arber, S. and Ginn, J. (1991) *Gender and Later Life: A Sociological Analysis of Resources and Constraints*. London, Sage.

Archibald, C. (1996) Home and away: people with dementia and their carers, in Stalker, K. (ed.) *Developments in Short-term Care: Breaks and Opportunities*. London, Jessica Kingsley, pp. 112–35.

Baillon, S., Scothern, G., Neville, P.G. and Boyle, A. (1996) Factors that contribute to stress in care staff in residential homes for the elderly. *International Journal of Geriatric Psychiatry*, **11**:219–26.

Brodaty, H. and Gresham, M. (1992) Prescribing residential respite care for dementia – effects, side-effects, indications and dosage. *International Journal of Geriatric Psychiatry*, **7**:357–62.

Burdz, M.P., Eaton, W.O. and Bond, J.P. (1988) Effect of respite care on dementia and nondementia patients and their caregivers. *Psychology and Aging*, **3**:38–42.

Challis, D., Darton, R., Johnson, L. et al. (1995) *Care Management and Health Care of Older People*. Aldershot, Arena.

Darnell, A., Davies, I., Pegram, M. et al. (1996) Taking a break or respite services for adults with learning disabilities, in Stalker, K. (ed.) *Developments in Short-term Care: Breaks and Opportunities*. London, Jessica Kingsley. pp. 24–34.

De Largy, J. (1957) Six weeks in – six weeks out: a geriatric hospital service for rehabilitating the aged and relieving their carers. *Lancet*, 23 February, 418–19.

Department of Health (1995) NHS Responsibilities for Meeting Continuing Health Care Needs. HSG(95) 8/ LAC (95) 5. NHS Executive, Department of Health, Leeds.

Goldberg, D. And Williams, P. (1988) *A User's Guide to the General Health Questionnaire*. Windsor: National Federation of Educational Research.

Henwood, M., Wistow, G. and Robinson, J. (1996) Halfway there? Policy, politics and outcomes in community care. *Journal of Social Policy and Administration*, **30**:39–53.

Kosloski, K. and Montgomery, R.J.V. (1995) The impact of respite use on nursing home placement. *Gerontologist*, **35**:67–74.

Levin, E., Moriarty, J. and Gorbach, P. (1994) *Better for the Break*. London, HMSO.

Levin, E., Sinclair, I. and Gorbach, P. (1989) *Families, Services and Confusion in Old Age*. Aldershot, Avebury.

Melzer, D. (1990) An evaluation of a respite care unit for elderly people with dementia: framework and some results. *Health Trends*, **22**:64–7.

Montgomery, R.J.V. and Borgatta, E.F. (1989) The effects of alternative support strategies on family caregiving. *Gerontologist*, **29**:457–64.

Oswin, M. (1991) *They Keep Going Away: A Critical Study of Short-term Residential Care. Services for Children with Learning Difficulties*, 2nd edn. London, King Edward's Hospital Fund for London.

Pattie, A.H. and Gilleard, C.J. (1979) *Manual of the Clifton Assessment Procedures for the Elderly*. Kent, Hodder & Stoughton.

Petch, A. (1996) Cairdeas House: developing good practice in short breaks for individuals with mental health problems, in Stalker, K. (ed.) *Developments in Short-term Care: Breaks and Opportunities*. London, Jessica Kingsley, pp. 136–54.

Qureshi, H. (1992) Young adults with learning difficulties and behaviour problems: parents views of services in the community. *Social Work and Social Sciences Review*, **3**(2):104–23.

Qureshi, H. (1993) Impact on families: young adults with learning disability who show challenging behaviour, in Kiernan, C. (ed.) *Research to Practice:*

Learning Disabilities and Challenging Behaviour. Kidderminster, British Institute of Mental Handicap, pp. 89–115.

Qureshi, H. and Nocon, A. (1996) *Report on Expert Seminars on Routine Outcome Measurement in the Personal Social Services.* York, Social Policy Research Unit.

Qureshi, H. and Walker, A. (1989) *The Caring Relationship.* Basingstoke, Macmillan.

Ramsay, M., Winget, C. and Higginson, I. (1995) Review: Measures to determine the outcome of community services for people with dementia. *Age and Ageing,* **24**:73–83.

Robertson, A., Gilloran, A., McGlew, T. *et al.* (1995) Nurses' job satisfaction and the quality of care received by patients in psychogeriatric wards. *International Journal of Geriatric Psychiatry,* **10**:575–84.

Robinson, C. (1991) *Home and Away: Respite Care in the Community.* Birmingham, Venture Press.

Robinson, C. (1996) Breaks for disabled children, in Stalker, K. (ed.) *Developments in Short-term Care: Breaks and Opportunities.* London, Jessica Kingsley, pp. 83–94.

Robinson, C. and Stalker, K. (1993) Patterns of provision in respite care and the Children Act. *British Journal of Social Work,* **23**:45–63.

Scharlach, A. and Frenzel, C. (1986) An evaluation of institution-based respite care. *Gerontologist,* **26**:77–82.

Schulz, R. and Williamson, G.M. (1991) A two year longitudinal study of depression among Alzheimer's caregivers. *Psychology and Aging,* **6**:569–78.

Sheldon, J.H. (1948) The Social Medicine of Old Age. Report of an inquiry in Wolverhampton. London, Nuffield Foundation.

Social Services Inspectorate (1993) *Guidance on Standards for Short-term Breaks.* London, HMSO.

Stalker, K. (1996) Principles, policy and practice in short term care, in Stalker, K. (ed.) *Developments in Short-term Care: Breaks and Opportunities.* London, Jessica Kingsley, pp. 5–23.

Twigg, J. (1989) Models of carers: how do agencies conceptualise their relation with informal carers. *Journal of Social Policy,* **18**:53–66.

Twigg, J. (1992) Carers in the service system, in Twigg, J. *Carers: Research and Practice.* London, HMSO, pp. 59–93.

Twigg, J. and Atkin, K. (1994) *Carers Perceived: Policy and Practice in Informal Care.* Milton Keynes, Open University Press.

Twigg, J. and Atkin, K. (1995) Carers and services: factors mediating service provision. *Journal of Social Policy,* **24**:5–30.

Twigg, J., Atkin, K. and Perring, C. (1990) *Carers and Services: A Review of Research.* London, HMSO.

Townsend, P. (1963) *The Family Life of Old People.* Harmondsworth, Penguin.

7 'WE NEED THE BED' – CONTINUING CARE AND COMMUNITY CARE

Kathleen Jones

Continuing the theme of the indispensability of certain of the specific functions of residential institutions, this chapter and the next confront head on the issue of whether dying old people can be appropriately cared for in the 'community'. As noted in several previous chapters, the number of continuing care beds in NHS hospitals has been reduced dramatically. Professor Jones provides case examples of the inability of fragmented community services and poorly trained staff to adequately care for the dying and unequivocally concludes that the only way to ensure proper care for people in the last months of their lives is the provision of more – not less – continuing care beds in residential settings.

'Dying is a very dull, dreary affair,' Somerset Maugham told his nephew, 'and I advise you to have nothing to do with it' (Maugham, 1972, p. 233). In recent years, the NHS Trusts have taken very much the same attitude.

People do not die to schedule. The last phase of life can be short or protracted, and its course is often very difficult to predict. For health service administrators, forced to manage their own budgets and to calculate in terms of 'bed-days', this is inconvenient. Reluctant to take on open-ended commitments, they have increasingly adopted a policy of discharging patients for whom no further medical intervention is prescribed, regardless of the human consequences.

140

Not all such patients are dying, not all of them are very old, but increasing numbers of very old and very sick patients who do not have long to live are being sent out of hospital in spite of the fact that they need *continuous process nursing care*. Some of them live alone and have no relatives or friends able to look after them. Their needs cannot be met by the fragmented community services, which are able to offer only short visits and are often not available when most needed. Private nursing home care is very expensive and often unsuited to these patients.

The *Panorama* programme

A television documentary in November 1994 (*Panorama*, 1994) highlighted some of the problems, citing cases in which patients had suffered considerable distress on being returned to their own homes. One man in his late seventies was sent home, paralysed from the neck down. He could not walk, wash his hands, bath, dress or feed himself, or even get in and out of a wheelchair. His only 'carer' was a frail elderly wife who could not lift him. The hospital's decision was that he did not 'require any further treatment', but it was conceded that he did require a certain amount of 'care assistance', for which the NHS should be responsible. This was estimated at 11 per cent of a worker's time. Assuming that the worker did an 8-hour day, and allowing time for travelling from case to case, that would provide something like 35 minutes a day.

In another case, a very old man was discharged from hospital, carefully placed in a chair in his flat – and left alone. A neighbour found him there *3 days later*, filthy and starving.

Interviews on the programme with local authority social services staff in different authorities revealed a mass of high-risk cases with which they did not have the resources to deal. The services were simply overwhelmed, and administrators frankly acknowledged that they could not provide the level of care that was needed. Often they were not notified quickly enough of vulnerable people who urgently needed attention. Even when notification was made quickly, they did not have the staff to make the visits.

Interviews with the hospital doctors responsible for discharging these patients revealed some curiously defensive attitudes (which may not have been sustained in private, away from the television cameras). One consultant took the view that, if there was no possibility of 'useful further recovery', the hospital had completed its task. What happened afterwards was not the concern of the NHS Trust. A second embarked on a semantic argument – 'What do you mean by ill?' Viewers were given to understand that if a patient could not be given medical treatment, he or she was not 'ill' but merely dying. Two more had clearly been taught by lecturers who enjoyed the use of diagrams. One said of a patient, 'He has reached a plateau', leaving viewers with a mental picture of the entire human race going downhill and occasionally pausing on the way down. The other sketched a semi-circle in the air, suggesting 'Perhaps he's at the extreme end of a spectrum'.

An NHS manager interviewed next was well versed in the policy of discharging patients who were no longer of interest to the medical profession. He said, 'We have to make hard-headed management decisions', and talked of setting priorities. It was evident that the condition of old and sick patients on discharge was of no interest to him – that was somebody else's problem. Last, the Secretary of State (then Virginia Bottomley) appeared on the programme. She acknowledged that there were problems and said that they were due to something called 'The Interface', a term she repeated several times. One wonders how many of her listeners knew what it meant. 'Social services', viewers were told, 'have a great deal more money'. Things could go wrong, but this only happened in 'a minority of cases'; 'It is quite important to distinguish between individual cases where something goes wrong, and the majority of cases... we have to learn from our problems.'

Three months later, the Department of Health issued new guidelines for hospitals and local authorities, to deal with the problems of the Interface.

The guidelines

The White Paper NHS *Responsibilities for Meeting Continuing Health Needs* (Department of Health, 1995) states that the arrangement and funding of services to meet continuing needs are 'an integral part of the responsibilities of the NHS' (clause 1), but that local authorities also have responsibilities for arranging and funding services to meet people's needs for continuing care, and collaboration is needed. There is nothing very new in this. The problem of continuity of care and the need to ensure collaboration between the different authorities involved has figured in many government reports since the inception of the NHS. Books have been written on the subject, conferences have been held, commissions and committees have sat and deliberated; and what none of them has been able to tell us is how this desirable degree of

working together is to be achieved between bodies whose organisational imperatives are so different and whose financial interests are
totally opposed.

The guidelines go on to spell out carefully the procedure for 'Hospital
Discharge Arrangements for People with Continuing Health Needs'
(clauses 16–24). The ultimate responsibility rests with the medical
consultant, but he is required to take into account 'an appropriate
multidisciplinary assessment of the patient's needs', arrived at after
consultation with social services staff. The arrangement should take
account of the views and wishes of the patient and the family or carer if
any. The patient may be judged to require 'continuing in-patient care
arranged and funded by the NHS' for any one of four reasons:

1. the need for 'on-going and regular clinical supervision' – usually
    once a week or more frequently;
2. the 'complexity, nature or intensity' of the patient's medical,
    nursing or other clinical needs;
3. the need for 'frequent or easily predictable interventions';
4. the fact that the prognosis is such that he or she is 'likely to die in
    the very near future, and discharge from the NHS would be
    inappropriate'.

Where a patient meets these eligibility criteria, and there is not a
hospital bed available, the NHS may meet the cost in another hospital or
a private nursing home. Hospital authorities are to provide 'simple
written information' about hospital discharge, and staff are to ensure
that 'patients, their families and any carers' have the necessary information to make key decisions. Social services staff are to provide written
details of the likely cost to the patient of any option that he or she is
asked to consider, including details of social security benefits payable
(clause 25). Patients who opt to go into nursing homes have the right to
decide which nursing home they go to and also the right to refuse to go
into a nursing home at all. If they refuse, they may be discharged to
their own homes, provided with 'a package of care' and charged for the
'social element' in care by the social services department.

There is a final safeguard; before 'such a discharge' (which must
mean one against the patient's will) is implemented, there is an appeals
procedure (clause 30). A patient, a family member or a carer has the
right to ask the health authority to review its decision, and the health
authority must reply in writing, usually within 2 weeks. This will
usually involve the advice of an independent panel. The double use of
'usually' suggests that these procedures will not necessarily be

followed, and the guidelines do not specify how the panels are to be formed. They do not have a legal status.

Reactions to the guidelines

A junior health minister introduced the document with the statement that 'NHS responsibility for care really does run from the cradle to the grave'. The *Independent* was unconvinced. Its headline on the new Guidelines was exactly the reverse: 'NHS guide ends free cradle-to-grave treatment'. The view expressed in the headline was attributed to a representative of the British Medical Association. The President of the Association of Directors of Social Services was cautious, predicting only that there would be local variations in interpretation. On the whole, most of those asked to give an opinion were cautious, praising the greater clarity offered by the guidelines but reserving judgement on how they would operate in practice. Nobody asked the people who would actually have to operate them – the harassed medical staff told by the consultant to 'clear four beds by tomorrow morning' for patients with more urgent needs; the hospital social workers given the unenviable task of explaining this maze of possibilities to very sick patients or distressed relatives; the district nurses, aware that they can make only very rapid interventions, because of the need to hurry on to the next case; the care managers struggling to cover an impossible number of tasks with a largely untrained workforce; the care workers, facing a multiplicity of demands, many of them well beyond their capacity to meet. And, of course, nobody asked the patients or their relatives.

Relatives may be distressed and confused. They may not grasp regulations and official procedures very readily. Some patients may have no relatives in the locality. In these days of scattered families, it is by no means unusual for old people living alone to have no kin within reach. Three cases illustrate the kinds of problems that can arise in practice.

Alice W was a tiny, bewildered 85-year-old, so thin that the bones stood out through her parchment-coloured flesh. She lived alone. She said that she had no relatives and no friends, and she did not know her neighbours, who were new and noisy. She had not bothered to eat, and, when she was taken into hospital, she was near starvation. Three weeks of vitamins and food supplements improved her condition to the point at which discharge was considered appropriate. The services swung into action. The occupational therapist took her to her flat to see if she could manage the stairs, get out of bed and walk to the toilet, and decided that she could. The hospital social worker explained about pensions and allowances. A telephone was installed, with an emergency button. Meals on Wheels were arranged. A care worker was engaged through a private agency.

On paper, everything was in place, but when I visited her a week later, Alice was again without food, and none of the arrangements worked as prescribed. She said that her problems had started even before she left the hospital. Nobody told her how to get home when she left the ward. The hospital was in an unfamiliar part of town. She went down to the entrance hall and hung about there for quite a time before a friendly porter telephoned for a taxi. She was not used to taking taxis and was frightened that she would not have enough money to pay for it. When she reached her flat, it was cold, and she had no food. She went out and bought some buns, and then went to bed. She did not understand the telephone and was frightened to use the emergency button. She had sent the care worker away, because she did not know how much she would cost and she did not like having strangers 'interfering'. She was not taking Meals on Wheels: 'You've got to be ready at the door when they come, with the money in your hand, they won't wait, and it's all paying out.' She had not seen her doctor. She did not feel well enough to go to the surgery, and he did not like making home visits.

While I was with Alice, offering to do her shopping and run her to the doctor, her first official visitor arrived. She was aged about 25, introduced herself as 'Debbie', and neglected to say what agency she had come from. She had a clip-board and a questionnaire. Ignoring the fact that Alice had another visitor, she sailed straight into a questionnaire:

'On what date were you discharged from hospital, Alice?'

'I don't know. Was it the Monday or the Tuesday... .'

'At what time did you arrive home?'

'Oh, it would be some time in the afternoon – or was it the morning? I get a bit muddled, you see'.

'Were you satisfied with your treatment in hospital?'

'Oh yes, the nurses were lovely'.

A tick in the box marked 'Very Satisfied'.

'And are you satisfied with your care since you returned to your own home?'

'Oh yes.' Alice said nervously.

Another tick at the positive end of the Likert Scale.

Presumably, this is the current status of the science of quality control. It was clear that Debbie, wherever she came from, did not understand even the rudiments of social work or research interviewing. She embarked on the questionnaire 'cold' and went straight through the preset questions without explanation. There were no questions about how Alice got home from hospital, whether she was in touch with her GP, whether she was eating properly, or whether she had friends or neighbours who helped her. No attempt was made to check the adequacy of the services provided. All the questions were at the level of 'Are you happy about... ?' or 'Are you satisfied with... ?' They were what the Latin primers call 'nonne' questions, expecting the answer 'Yes'. This is a perversion of respectable social science methodology.

When Debbie had made the final tick, she recited mechanically 'Thank you very much for your time' and departed. Alice had plenty of time. What she needed was practical action. Presumably, the paper record piles up and protects somebody's job somewhere. 'Cheek,' said Alice, stung into a febrile indignation, 'Coming in here and asking me all those daft questions. And calling me Alice. I never saw her before, Debbie indeed'.

Alice was soon back in hospital. After a further 3 weeks of vitamins and food supplements, she was again told that she must leave, but the consultant did not think that she was fit to go back to her flat: she would have to go into a nursing home. People came to explain about the nursing home, but Alice did not know where it was, what it would be like or how it would be paid for. Somebody took her flat key out of her purse, and she did not know what was happening to her possessions. She grew increasingly confused and disoriented, and physically weaker. Before anything could be finally arranged, she died in hospital.

'Community care' had been defined as a set of procedures, mechanically carried out. They manifestly did not meet Alice's needs. Workers did not understand that someone of her age and social background was not used to taxis, telephones and nursing homes. They did not understand that an old lady who has been making ends meet on a tiny pension for years might be frightened of spending money and not know how to handle it, unless the cash were actually on the table in front of her. Paper figures and talks about an allowance were simply meaningless to Alice. Of course, this is an extreme case: Alice was lost in a world where people assumed that she had a social competence she had never possessed and could not learn. Another case, however, illustrates what can happen even to people who are normally highly competent at running their own lives and who are well able to pay for care.

Henry G was a retired accountant who had made prudent provision for his old age after his wife died. When he could no longer live alone, he moved to a small hotel in Torquay and lived there very comfortably for some years. He was 86 when he developed heart problems and was admitted to hospital. His only sister, aged 81, came down from Scotland to be with him and was greeted with the information that the hospital could not keep him 'because he might live for some time'. She was asked to move him elsewhere as soon as possible. She was given a list of nursing homes in the vicinity and advised to visit them: she spent most of the next 2 weeks visiting nursing homes. Some were unsuitable for a man in a terminal condition. Some could not take him at short notice. Some were not keen to take a dying patient (it looks bad in the statistics). During that time, the consultant tried three times to discharge Henry and was only prevented by a ward sister who stood at the end of the bed and said flatly, 'My patient is not fit to be discharged.' Then, to everybody's relief, Henry died. His last few days of life were clouded by the knowledge that the hospital was trying to get rid of him, and his sister's last contacts with him were cut short by the problem of trying to find a nursing home. Henry had managed his own retirement admirably until his final breakdown. He could have paid for any kind of care – but what he needed was not available, even at a price.

Other problems of nursing home care are illustrated by a third case. Joe M had been in hospital continuously for over 4 months. He had been an army sergeant in the Second World War, an old campaigner, with plenty of experience in how to survive, but at the age of 79, with only one lung, a weak heart and a malfunctioning liver, he was fighting his last battle. The prognosis when he was admitted was that he would live for only a few weeks. He endured a battery of medical tests and scans, two operations and a long period of dialysis. He wanted to be left alone to die quietly, but it seemed that the doctors were determined to go on treating him, to justify the fact that he was still in hospital. At the end of 4 months, he was still alive and did not need further dialysis. It was decided that no more could be done in the way of treatment and that, since he lived alone, he was unfit to go home. A social worker took him by taxi to see three nursing homes after explaining that he would be expected to pay about £400 a week for his care. The visits took most of a day, and Joe, who was still very weak, found them distressing and exhausting. He had always lived very frugally: £400 was as much as he normally spent in a month, and he was afraid that his savings would soon disappear. He was shrewd enough in assessing what he would be offered for his money, and he did not like what he saw. At one home, he asked to see the daily menu and was told there was no menu – food was standard, and there were no alternatives. At another, it was suggested (although he was in a wheelchair) that he might help out by working in the garden – 'What me, when I'm paying £400 a week?' He found all three very depressing: 'the old men were just sitting round the wall'. When he got back thankfully into his hospital bed, he flatly refused to be moved to any of them. 'I'm a British citizen,' he said, 'I fought in the War, and I paid my taxes. Go into one of those places and pay £400 a week for it? Not likely.' Most of the doctors and nurses said 'Good for you, Joe.'

The hospital managed to find him a bed for another fortnight, but he still did not die. Eventually, it was decided that he really must be discharged. The guidelines had been in operation for over 8 months, but the appeals procedure did not seem to be operating. If it was, nobody told Joe about it, and he was sent home very quickly once the decision was made. He went to his own flat after being warned that he would be provided with a 'package of care' and expected to pay for it. His GP visited and gave him 3 weeks at most to live. The district nurse visited. Social services provided a young care assistant twice a day, but she only stayed for a short time on each visit and expected Joe to tell her what to do. He was too ill to know or care. She was willing enough but clearly had no experience of terminal nursing. Joe stayed in bed, too weak to get up and answer the front door. He had to leave the door unlocked, which worried him, because 'anybody could get in, not that I've got much to steal. But you do hear of such awful cases... ' There was another one in the local paper that night – an elderly pensioner robbed and beaten up.

Social services did their best. They increased the visits by the care assistant to three a day and sent a relief worker in at the weekends, but there was a crisis over a Bank Holiday, when nobody was available. Joe collapsed and was found on the floor, unconscious. His GP could not secure a hospital bed for him. At last he was persuaded, much against his will, to go into a nursing home.

The nursing home was a new one, with over 800 beds. The buildings were impressive, the furnishing were excellent, and the paintwork was glossy. Joe, who was a proud and reserved man, was assured that he could have a room to himself. He expected to stay in it and to be nursed, but when I called to see him, he was sitting, silent and mutinous, in a room with all the other old men. They were supposed to be watching Donald Duck on the television, but each was in a world of his own. The nurse in charge said, 'They're better out of bed' and 'They're often fretful at first, but they soon settle down.' I called again, 2 days later. Joe was still in the communal lounge, leaning back exhausted in a wheelchair. A care assistant was trying to make him play bingo. When I asked to see the matron and told her of the GP's prognosis, she said, 'Oh, I don't think he's *ill*, is he? We haven't been told that he's *ill*'. Joe would not talk about the situation – he seemed frozen with weakness and apathy; but that afternoon he discharged himself and was taken home again.

Within 24 hours, he collapsed once more, and his harassed GP found a solution; the fact that Joe was within hours of death was not enough to get him a hospital bed, so he made a new diagnosis – Joe was suffering from anaemia, a treatable condition. The ward sister recognised the situation at once. She had probably encountered it many times. She said, 'All we can do is to make him comfortable.' He drifted into a coma and died the following day.

Joe had spent most of his long life in the belief that *sick people went into hospital*. He did not understand a world in which the hospital had become *a place where medical intervention was carried out*. He knew nothing about nursing homes and did not like what he saw. Although some of the staff had nursing qualifications (a local authority requirement), the home was geared not to the treatment of very sick people but to the occupation of the long-term disabled; but if it was not a medical establishment, neither was it the kind of residential home that social services used to run. It was clear that the staff, although well intentioned, had no training of any kind in residential care or the preservation of the residents' personal identities. They knew nothing of Joe's medical record or his personal needs, and it was not a home in any sense of the word: it was a large institution run by a financial syndicate for profit. Perhaps the local authority inspectors were impressed by the white paint, the expensive curtains, the excellent fire precautions and the size of the car park; but who trains the inspectors?

The Interface

Presumably Alice, Henry and Joe (three very different people known to the writer personally over the 18 months prior to writing this chapter) were all 'at the end of the spectrum'. Although the situation has become more acute in recent years, the problems of the Interface are of long standing. They arise chiefly from three factors: the increased expectation of life, which means that there are more very old people in need of care than in previous generations; the low prestige of medicine for the dying – death is often seen as a medical failure rather than an inevitable stage in human existence; and the steady move from statutory responsibility for health and welfare services to the philosophy of 'market forces' (Plant, 1985).

Even in the early days of the NHS, its tripartite structure caused problems in securing continuity of care. The situation was not too acute as long as the Interface was only a matter of argument between hospitals and local authorities, but the National Health Service and Community Care Act of 1990 introduced three highly significant policy changes. First, there was the shift to financially autonomous Hospital Trusts, which, responsible for their own budgets, could not afford open-ended commitments to individual patients. Second, the duties of local authorities to provide accommodation for 'aged and infirm persons' were amended. 'Infirmity' was replaced by 'illness' and 'disability', thus giving the hospital authorities a greater freedom to discharge very sick people. Third, nursing care was to be provided by 'a voluntary organization or other person managing premises'. Local authorities had been forced to close their own residential homes and to rely on other provision, largely in the private sector.

When this policy was first introduced in the 1980s, many of the private homes opened were small establishments, run by nurses on a domestic pattern, but costs were high and regulations stringent. Increasingly, they have been replaced by much larger establishments run by financial syndicates primarily interested in profits.The residents may receive retirement pension and Disability Living Allowance, but they have to pay the rest of the cost until their own resources are exhausted down to a specified minimum. Until the 1995 November Budget, individuals were liable for the full cost until they had £8,000 left and part of the cost until they had only £3,000 left. These amounts have now been increased to £15,000 and £9,000 respectively. No doubt this sounds generous to the many people who do not possess anything like these sums. The catch is that the assessment includes all the resident's resources, including his or her home. People of moderate means in their seventies and eighties now face the prospect that, if they do not die quickly when their time comes, their savings and their homes, secured after decades of careful management and mortgage payments, will be swallowed up in large nursing home bills. Some are concerned that the inheritance they had hoped to leave to their children will be exhausted. Others worry that, after a lifetime of independence, they will see their homes broken up, run out of funds and become a charge on the state. The worst feature is the loss of personal control. After a lifetime of independence, they face the prospect of being shunted from place to place like an inconvenient parcel at the time when they most need stability and reassurance .

Economists and financiers now advise people to take out their own private health insurance, but people who are elderly now cannot take out insurance against a risk they never expected to have to face. During their working lives, the health service provided care for terminally ill patients. Insurance policies, even if they were available, would be too expensive now that they are living on pensions. But of course the insurance policies are not available. Even people now in their twenties and thirties cannot take out adequate insurance against the risks of a long period of physical dependency. The insurance companies are, understandably, not prepared to write blank cheques. Benefits are always time-limited.

What can be done?

It is necessary to be realistic. The time when social scientists could end the analysis of a social problem with a simple prescription for 'more resources' are long past. Medical science has increased the expectation of life, finding cures for the acute diseases of middle age (which used to carry people off relatively quickly), thus ensuring that more will reach the state not merely of chronic illness, but of final physical breakdown – a state in which the syndrome is so complex that the question of diagnosis becomes almost academic. Doubtless it will go on doing so, but the problems cannot be solved by talk about the Interface or budgetary concessions. Below are some suggestions.

First, the guidelines must be taken seriously and not remain at the level of central government rhetoric. Patients should be told clearly about the appeals procedure and given time to operate it before they are bundled out of the wards. All three of the patients whose cases have been discussed were 'likely to die in the very near future'. Perhaps there might be room for argument in individual cases over the uncertainties of 'likely to die' and the length of 'the very near future' (was that deliberately vague drafting by the Department of Health?), but all three certainly required continuous nursing care of a kind which they could not be given in the community.

Health service administrators may argue that they are severely restricted for money; some (although by no means all) members of the medical profession may argue for triage – concentrating their skills on the living rather than the half dead; but how much needless and expensive technological treatment is being performed on patients like Joe, who really need only to be 'made comfortable', just to justify their continued stay in hospital? Of course, this is a matter for medical judgement in individual cases, but the need for nursing care of such patients should be recognised in its own right – and not as a mere adjunct to medical technology.

Second, old and sick people whose condition is probably terminal, and who live alone, are at special risk. If they are discharged to their own homes and have no immediate relatives, the alarm bells should start ringing. Ward staff should ensure that they can get home, and the social services department should be notified by telephone or fax to visit on the same day. This need not involve a visit by a social worker: a care assistant could ensure that there is food available and that there is heating if the house or flat is cold. The health care team should be notified as a similar matter of urgency.

Third, social workers and care assistants need training in dealing with confused and very sick old people like Alice, for whom rational explanation based on the assumptions of a younger generation are not enough. Some of them simply do not understand the modern world of telephones, taxis and paper money transactions. Workers need to ask the commonsense questions – What's in your pantry or refrigerator?, Who does your shopping?, Have you got toilet paper, a hot water-bottle, tea in the tea-caddy?, Can you get to the doctor? – rather than filling in agency-orientated questionnaires by rote.

Fourth, the staff of private sector nursing homes need training in residential care – and in the pathologies of institutional care. It was painfully obvious that none of the staff in Joe's home had ever heard of Goffman and 'batch living'. They were good people, doing their best, but has 35 years of post-Goffman teaching in residential care simply disappeared because the responsibilities have been handed over to the private sector?

Fifth, local authority inspectors may need additional training, too. It is not enough to look at physical provision in homes: they should be capable of assessing the quality of care, and of improving it by advice and encouragement. The knowledge of how to do this has not been entirely lost. It is widely practised in the hospice movement, in which the last phase of life is treated as 'quality time', meaningful in its own right, and with sensitivity to individual needs and preferences. The contrast between this kind of good, voluntary care and the muddled and inadequate care of patients caught in the trap of the Interface is acute.

Sixth, we need to find a national solution to the 'blank cheque' problem – how to provide financial cover for the risks of a long terminal illness. If this cannot be provided out of general taxation, and the insurance companies do not find it financially viable, government must find a better answer. One solution would be to limit the individual's responsibility in terms of time as well by cash limits. Many people would be willing to pay for insurance against the necessity of long-term care for themselves for a year, perhaps 2 years; and the insurance companies might well be able to work out suitable terms. For nearly all, that would be enough. The problem lies in the uncertainty that one might be one of the small minority for whom the final phase is a long one. If there was an agreed period after which the state would provide full coverage, individuals would be encouraged to make their own provision up to that time.

Finally, whether in the health service or in the private sector, however financed, we need units in which very old, very sick people can be *nursed* and not treated like the younger disabled. Dying is a process that happens to everyone in time, and the denial of this process is one of the new institutional pathologies. Very few people can want to go through it playing bingo.

Most of these suggestions are palliative, suggested in a social context in which public sector provision is no longer backed by political will, as it was in the days of the 'welfare consensus' and at a time when the whole of the European Community is devoted to the task of reducing public expenditure at all costs. Some social costs are simply too great. Some of us would prefer to see decent, civilised provision made for the dying, even if it means a penny or two on the income tax.

Note: the three cases cited in this paper occurred in different localities, names and identifying details have been changed.

References

Department of Health (1995) *NHS Responsibilities for Meeting Continuing Health Needs*, HSG (95) 8, LAC (95) 5 February 1995. HMSO, London.

Maugham, R. (1972) *Escape from the Shadows*. London, Hodder.

Panorama, BBC 1 7 November, 1994.

Plant, R. (1985) The very idea of welfare, in Bean, P., Ferris, J. and Whynes, D. (eds) *In Defence of Welfare*. London, Tavistock, pp. 3–30.

8 Death and Dying in Residential Homes for Older People

Yvonne Shemmings

In this chapter, Yvonne Shemmings explores further the specific functions of residential institutions. The previous chapter discussed the role of continuing care for dying old people in relation to the impact of community care policy on the provision of such care within the NHS. Seventy-one per cent of all deaths now occur in residential institutions; partly as a result of the redefinition of the role of medical institutions within the reforms of community care, residential homes are increasingly fulfilling this caring function. The marginalisation and neglect of residential institutions resulting from the dualistic conception of 'residential care is bad, community care is good' has contributed to the staff of such homes being ill prepared for this daunting task. This chapter explores the nature of the denial of death in our society, its consequent sequestration in residential institutions and the ways in which the demands this poses can be met in best practice within them.

Although many people will say that they would prefer to 'die at home', what they often go on to say is that they would prefer to 'die with their loved ones around them', failing which they might accept, or tolerate, being cared for by sensitive adults (even though not related to them). Most people would not prefer to die at home if this meant being cold, lonely and forgotten. And even if loved ones are around, it is difficult for dying people to find peace if they feel that their decline is tearing apart those for whom they most care.

154

In this chapter, I argue that modern society will be unwilling to provide the resources for *older* people to die at home, and that, as a consequence, there will be an increasing demand for residential care, but now as a place to end one's life. Thus a dilemma is exposed: to give a dying person what he or she most wants and needs – one's presence and one's time – inevitably means more and better prepared staff. Failure to provide such caring people is likely to result in death and dying becoming an essentially lonely and even terrifying experience for residents. Professionals in social care often talk about a resident's 'quality of life'; it is argued here that residents' 'quality of life', *and* their 'quality of death and dying', will be significantly affected if those charged with their care are not prepared physically and psychologically. This is the central challenge for residential homes if they are to have a role in the provision of better care to people as they come to the end of their life, a role which I believe staff can and should perform.

Ann Cartwright (1991) claimed that 'the evidence suggests that because of their age and frailty those living in residential homes will have needed more care during the last year of their lives than other people who have died' (p. 634), and she had already concluded, 'Increasingly, the quality of life during the year before death is going to depend upon the attributes of residential homes and their staff' (p. 627). Various statistics support her arguments:

> By the mid-1960s, two thirds of all deaths in the United Kingdom occurred in hospitals or other places caring for the sick, and by 1989 this had risen to 71% with only 23% of home deaths [p. 8].... Currently, 12–15% of all deaths occur in residential or nursing homes, a figure that is likely to rise. [p. 17] (Field and James, 1993)

During 1994 and 1995 I studied in depth the experiences of 20 staff in residential homes for older people. One of the reasons for doing this research was that 'There is very little literature and even less research on this theme. Though death is more readily discussed, very little has been written on death and dying within residential and nursing home settings' (Counsel and Care, 1995, p. 8). One key implication can be crystallised from my research, and it relates specifically to the theme of this book: because older people entering residential homes are nowadays more frail than ever before, the relationship between attachment and loss is likely to become more complicated for staff. The end of life is discussed openly in hospices; it is my view that staff and residents in residential homes for older people also should be encouraged to talk more about death and dying.

The role of residential care workers has shifted from simply assisting residents to something barely distinguishable from nursing care. This shift is not entirely the result of residents becoming more physically dependent, with staff needing physically to lift and feed them; it stems also from the diversity of situations which care staff encounter in residential homes. This is something that is often not acknowledged. When on duty, staff are required to make constant adjustments according to the situation in which they find themselves with residents. Whilst some are extremely frail physically, others may hit staff or other residents; others may call out incessantly and seem to be quite unaware of their behaviour. Many seem disorientated, and they may say repeatedly that they want to return home, and arguably many have little or no conception any more of what that 'home' means to them. They may be unaware of why they are living in residential care. It is against this backdrop that residential workers care for vulnerable people who are dying. My research set out to explore the tensions and dilemmas for care assistants, some of which emerge in the following two extracts:

> Mary is a young care assistant. Three years ago she returned home and found her fiancé dead, lying in bed. He had taken an overdose of his medication, prescribed for depression. In her job, Mary has to cope with her feelings when she hears people in their eighties and nineties crying with pain, saying that they want to die, or listen to people distressed and lost in their confusion. She says she seeks peace in the faces of the residents when they have died to help lay to rest the ghost of her contorted fiancé. She is afraid that death is always distressing and full of pain. She likes to tend to residents immediately after they have died to make sure the relatives may see them looking peaceful. (Shemmings, 1996, p. 1)

> Alice walks down the corridor in answer to the sound of a buzzer from the lounge. John wanted to go to the toilet but was unable to wait. His clothes need changing. There are others too who need help to go to the toilet... a relative is waiting to see how his mother is... and all the while Jane is dying, alone, in her room. (Shemmings, 1996, pp. 1–2)

Death and dying: taboo... or not taboo?

Geoffrey Gorer was one of the first to observe that society is often fascinated with the idea of death. It was Gorer (1955) who described the saturation of images of death in the media as the 'pornography of death'. But, paradoxically, although there remains a fascination with death, many authors argue that a taboo also exists, especially regarding who should provide care to a dying person, in the sense that it is generally thought of as best left to the 'professionals'. This taboo is seen as being socially constructed and is borne out of society's fear of death and reluctance or inability to care physically for dying people within the family. Consequently, it is assumed that people prefer to die surrounded by professionals in a medical setting but not necessarily in a hospital (see Ariès, 1981).

Many of society's values are reflected in the care of the dying, and, as Philippe Ariès pointed out, it was the dislocation between the living and the dying that became culturally accepted, and thus the 'denial of death' followed (Ariès, 1974). However, as one would expect, 'death' and 'dying' are highly contested medical and social categories. Clive Seale, for example, takes issue with the idea that death is routinely 'denied'. His objection is that:

> In fact, calls to cease denying death and to resist 'medicalisation' have not gone unheard. Within the hospice movement psychological expertise is marshalled to ensure that death is anticipated, prepared for, and above all accompanied. (Seale, 1995, p. 377)

For Seale, the point is that 'hospitals appear not to offer opportunities for accompaniment' (p. 30). Other authors also disagree about the extent to which death is 'denied'. For example, many people, especially those in later life, have been socialised to think of death as occurring in an institution. In a culture in which health, wealth, intelligence and activity are valued highly and where sick, infirm, old and disabled people are marginalised, it is not surprising that, as Kearl (1989) points out, 'death has become an alien intruder, disrupting the satisfactions of the here and now'. Taking a contrary view, however, Blauner (1966) concluded that death in modern society is not taboo; rather, it is simply 'no big deal'. He argued that it is not forbidden but merely hidden.

Historically, a slow decline and controlled retreat into death was considered to be essential to the 'good' death. People prepared themselves for death through ritual and well-rehearsed customs. Nowadays, death and disease are to be conquered and fought at all costs. With people living longer, beyond their 'three score years and ten', the term 'post-mature death' has emerged to distinguish it from 'pre-mature death'. Post-mature death, however, conjures up visions of older people in some way outstaying their welcome. This, coupled with society's reluctance or inability to provide financially for its elders, leaves uncertain the likelihood of good care being available for very dependent older people who are dying in residential care. Moreover, moving into residential care is increasingly seen as a precursor to death, and, with the closure of hospital wards and health policies that allow admission only during the acute stage of an illness, those deemed to be chronically ill (which now includes people with cancer) are often discharged from hospital into residential care in their last days or hours of life.

Dying in institutions

The gradual withdrawal of the process of death from the family created a space that has been filled by medical institutions (see Kearl, 1989). Although concerned primarily with the preservation of life, hospitals are nevertheless accepted by society as places where death occurs; whereas hospices exist to combine medical treatment and palliative care, and to provide specialised counselling. The point is that, unlike most care assistants in residential homes, staff in hospitals and hospices are professionally trained, and many also have specific knowledge about the care and treatment of dying people.

It was the notion of a more human response to death and dying which first gave rise to the hospice movement and the more widespread development of bereavement counselling. However, the demand for the limited and very specialised resources afforded by the hospice movement ensures that only those considered to be the highest priority receive the service. It is rare for very old people to be transferred to a hospice from either their own home, a hospital or a residential home prior to death because a slow decline often prevents diagnosis of the terminal stage of their illness. However, although there is some evidence that older people close to death are more likely to 'accept' death (Hinton, 1972), they are likely nevertheless to have many hopes and fears – and nightmares or dreams – about which they would welcome an opportunity to talk. This tendency to assume that people accept death when older may mask a need to talk, and it may further indicate death 'denied'.

As stated already, staff in residential homes receive far less of the training and support which their colleagues in hospices enjoy, but although staff in medical institutions used to be more familiar with death among their patients than did staff in residential care homes, this is rapidly changing. Nowadays, residential homes provide more care than ever before to people who are dying. The line between what takes place in medical settings and in residential homes has become blurred. The latter have become places for the chronically sick, and, as such, 'home' can sometimes appear to bear little resemblance to the activities normally experienced in one's own home. In the past, for most people, entering a residential home did not raise the expectation of impending death; after all, it was a 'home'. People *live* in a home;

they *die* in hospices, hospitals or in nursing homes. But this is less true today; people do die in residential homes, and new residents often say that they think about this a lot. It is therefore confusing to staff and residents if, to use Peter Townsend's phrase (1964), it is not appreciated that the home may be their 'last refuge', or , as one of the interviewees put it, 'God's waiting room'.

In respect of the care assistant's routines and the constant coming and going of community nurses and doctors, residential homes have become more like a medical institution; but in respect of staff selection and training, there are major differences. Furthermore, staff wearing uniforms may lead to a false expectation of the home as being somewhere where medical and nursing expertise is freely available. Yet care assistants are neither doctors nor nurses. Also, through such symbols, wrong impressions may be given to both 'insiders' and 'outsiders' about the type of care that can be offered: medical practitioners and nurses, for example, often refer to residential homes as 'nursing homes'.

The nature of residential care is changing. Staff often say that they prefer to care for residents rather than see them admitted to hospital, even though they understand that much of their time will be spent solely on their individual care. Yet in doing so, they may be masking the personal and emotional cost to themselves. Also they know that to spend time with a dying person places a burden on the remaining staff which in turn affects the care given to other residents. Staff selection and recruitment takes little account of the need for a workforce capable of dealing with distressing situations, especially if the interview process does not address the applicant's ability to be with and care for dying people. Additionally, in-house training in residential care is usually scant and expensive to provide in terms of time and staff cover, the implications of which affect both residents and staff. Consequently, staff may feel ill equipped and unsupported in their task.

Death and dying in residential homes: messages from the study

My research comprised an intensive qualitative study into the experiences of staff who cared for dying residents (see Shemmings, 1996). Twenty staff were interviewed in five local authority residential homes. One interviewee was a home manager, one was an assistant manager and another occupied a relief manager's post. The remaining 17 were care assistants. A semi-structured interview schedule was used to explore a range of views and experiences. The interviews were tape-recorded.

Three main themes emerged: from the tapes, differences were noted between the *attitudes*, *feelings* and *actions* of those interviewed. Within these themes, they spoke at length about their attitudes to ageing, their religious beliefs, feelings of attachment to residents, feelings as a result of past losses in their own lives, and feelings when a resident approached the last stages of life. Finally, it was possible to see how the experiences of staff can be understood through their actions when caring for dying people.

The interviews contain many moving accounts. The strength and range of feelings capture many of the tensions and dilemmas for staff when caring for people who are dying. This is illustrated very simply by the different adjectives used to describe those feelings: 'awkwardness', 'grief', 'powerlessness', 'fear', 'pain', 'loss', 'guilt', sorrow', 'vulnerability', 'injustice' and 'loneliness'. Those interviewed did express more positive feelings – 'optimism', 'reconciliation', 'achievement', 'peacefulness', 'attachment' and 'reassurance' – but, perhaps not unexpectedly, these were heard far less frequently. A number of key messages emerged from the study including:

● The need for care workers to be with the dying person, to hold his or her hand, to pause for a while to say goodbye (even if only to the empty room afterwards) without feeling guilty that other residents are being ignored or neglected, and to attend the funeral.

● The need, after the person has died, to be able to talk to colleagues and receive support... or sometimes simply to be quiet and reflect.

● Although those interviewed believed that, broadly speaking, they knew how to *care* for a resident who was dying, they often felt at a loss to know what to *say* to the person about death and dying.

● They spoke candidly about their need to know that the sheer emotional pain and loss that they experienced every time a resident died was understood and appreciated – 'It's hard... it's so hard'. (Shemmings, 1996)

It is possible that residential homes could become less institutionalised as places in which to die because, even though its symbols and messages may confuse the 'outside' community, its residents and perhaps even its staff concerning its primary purpose, it may be more akin to dying at home, in one's own bed, surrounded by as many personal possessions as is feasible, than it is in other institutions in which death happens routinely.

If it is the case that residential homes have already become places where people die, as the main alternative to their own home, it is then perhaps not surprising to learn that staff caring for very dependent residents see many of them as they would members of their own family. One interviewee said, 'I view them as my own mother or father'. This can lead to resentment and anger towards those families who do not visit their relative in the home 'yet attend the funeral and weep'. This worker equated 'visiting' with 'caring' for the person and saw such residents as being sadder than those who had no family at all: 'There's so many excuses for not coming to see that person when they're alive – I feel really sad.' For residents, too, many staff become their substitute family, with a genuine reciprocity of interest being developed and shared: 'When my daughter got married, [one resident] said: "You must bring the photos."' One of the challenges for residential homes in the future is how to find ways of supporting staff when they form such attachments. Otherwise, how can residential workers be expected to cope with more loss and separation in 6 months than most of us feel in a lifetime? Failure to meet this challenge is likely to lead either to detached caring or increased stress for staff, or both. And it is precisely *because* care assistants in residential homes – more, it is argued, than their colleagues in hospices and hospitals – get to know the resident well that these dilemmas and challenges bubble to the surface so quickly.

The relationships developed between staff and residents may also serve to replicate eroded or lost traditions in society: by being with the person during the last days, hours and moments before death; when performing 'last offices' for the deceased; or by straightening them, washing them and preparing them for relatives to sit with prior to their removal by the undertakers.

Staff are sometimes even asked to fulfil the role of priest when people are dying. One person interviewed recalled a woman who was dying and who was particularly restless and distressed. Recognising that something out of the ordinary was worrying the resident, the worker asked if she needed to tell her something but that she would get a priest if she preferred. The resident declined the priest but told the worker that she felt very guilty about the way she had treated her own daughter as a child. The worker asked if she would like to tell her daughter herself, but the resident seemed happy to have confided her 'guilty' feelings to the care assistant. Having heard the worker say that she had done the right thing by confiding this to her, the resident then became calm, and soon afterwards she died. Without proper support and training, the weight of such confessions on the shoulders of a care assistant could be overwhelming.

Working with people who are dying demands considerable personal involvement (Saunders, 1965). For some staff, whilst attachment to residents is synonymous with 'good care', for others it is important for them not to become too involved because 'there is always another person to be cared for when others die'. As one care assistant put it, 'One dies, then it's on with the next one.' Another worker actively tried not to become involved with residents but concluded that 'you do try to keep neutral, but it is not always possible'. Fear of strong emotions prevented one care assistant becoming too involved emotionally in the lives of residents: 'You do not have to be emotionally involved with everybody – emotions, if they come out, can destroy the person.' Attachment is not, it seems, an automatic response in care work, although it is clear from many staff that they form very close relationships with some residents but, for understandable reasons, not everyone.

When it proves impossible for a member of staff to be with a resident at the time of death (perhaps because their shift had ended), almost everyone interviewed said that they felt moved to go into the deceased person's room. Some said they whisper a prayer; some just 'touch the bed' and say 'goodbye'. Others, however, felt that they had not truly said farewell unless and until they had attended the funeral (which it is not always possible to permit, due to staffing levels, sickness and so on).

It is clear from most of the literature that, if some people are deeply affected by loss, a process of bereavement is necessary for healthy psychological healing to take place. One care assistant acknowledged that she came into the work to reassure herself that some people do, in fact, die of 'old age', but peacefully, as distinct from the premature and painful death experienced by her own mother. Experience of personal loss was a recurring theme in the interviews. A sad testimony came from this same care assistant, who admitted to never having really come to terms with the death of her own mother. She gained a little comfort from the 'kisses and cuddles' she had with some residents, but the death of a resident to whom she had been particularly close had rekindled strong feelings of loss and she described herself as being 'devastated... I cried for weeks'. And then, tearfully, she added that she 'would never get that attached again'.

At times, the resilience of staff seems remarkable; it this resilience which will be increasingly called upon, both if existing residents become even more frail, and are not moved to hospital, or if new residents arrive in the home, either from hospital or the community, who need very high levels of care. One care assistant was horrified at the condition in which some people came into the home in which she worked. She said that one person had arrived in an ambulance from hospital virtually comatose and requiring constant care and attention in bed in what proved to be the last hours of her life:

> They actually seem to come in dying. It looks as if the hospital needs a bed, and they actually come into us dying!... . Sometimes they've lasted two weeks here, sometimes just one night – which is very wrong – somewhere along the line there has been a breakdown.

The same worker expressed a sense of injustice that staff were subjected to the difficulties inherent in caring for a very sick person: 'It puts a lot of pressure on us. You start to take it within your stride. Whether that's a good thing or not, I don't know.' This was the crux of the matter for many staff, few of whom were trained in the specialised care of frail and dying people (and I am not thinking primarily of their 'physical' care).

The stresses on staff are reflected in the next excerpt, expressed by one care assistant who regretted that there was not enough time available to develop the sort of relationship that she would ideally prefer to establish with residents:

> I feel reasonably close, but it boils down to the fact that really we do not get time for one-to-one. That is a frustration of this job: you don't get time to sit and just chat and talk things through. I would prefer to work on a more personal level.

However, it is not simply that staff would like to enhance relationships. They are also acutely aware that, while they are assisting someone to the toilet or attending to the personal needs of one resident, another may be alone, dying, in their room. The tension created by oscillating between the needs of so many people has a profound effect on a worker's sense of job satisfaction. It is doubtful that the following comments will be the norm in future if it is not recognised that to care for elderly people at the end of their lives needs all the love, compassion, time and commitment of their carers. If *their* needs are not acknowledged, I believe that staff will bend to the weight of the institution, and then the quality of both life *and* death, will be sacrificed:

> You feel satisfaction in a job well done – knowing you have done a good job and that someone has benefited from me being in this building. It does make a difference.

> If you have known someone they have become part of you, and you go back to the days when they were admitted. You think, 'I've got a personal responsibility for others' happiness', and you hope to have made the last months or years happy for them.

When death is an accepted and publicly acknowledged feature of the institution in which it occurs, staff may begin to feel clearer about their role in this respect. However, unlike the situation in hospices and hospitals, for example, the role for workers in residential homes when caring for dying people is far less clearly defined. As we have seen, much of the confusion, and the tension and dilemma, surrounds the complex areas of attachment, separation and loss. There are lessons here, too, which can be applied to community workers. For example, higher dependency creates a need for more intimate physical care. Similarly, greater mental frailty can create the need for field and domiciliary workers to 'protect' service users, which can in turn lead to a strong bond developing between the two; thus attachments are formed with all their inherent peaks and troughs. Staff may be seduced by the symbols and routines of the home, which may affect how they perceive their task. Taking their responsibilities very seriously, they become attached to those for whom they care. And the closer staff become to those with whom they work, the harder it is emotionally for the worker when the resident dies.

Conclusion

As we have seen, Clive Seale (1995) stresses the need for dying people to be 'accompanied' during the last stages of life. A publication by Counsel and Care in May 1995 called *Last Rights* contains this powerful statement:

> Death is rarely joyful, and dying in a home can be a particularly melancholy business. Retreating from one's own home and loved ones to an anonymous establishment is a poor prelude to the last days of life, a time when almost everyone wants to be surrounded by familiar sights and sounds and by loving and well remembered friends and relatives. To meet one's end without such comfort is the ultimate loneliness. (Counsel and Care, 1995, p. 1)

One of the interviewees with whom I spoke said something similar: 'They just need to know they have got a friend – that someone cares – especially if they have no relations, and especially if they are dying – just to know someone is there' (Shemmings, 1996, p. 56). For residential homes to offer such comfort – such 'accompaniment' – there would need to be an open acknowledgement that many of those who enter residential care will die there. For the 'institution' to become a 'home', staff will need support and training similar to those working in other places where death occurs. For this to happen in residential homes, it will mean that the subject of death and dying can no longer be buried.

References

Ariès, P. (1974) *Western Attitudes Toward Death: From the Middle Ages to the Present*. Baltimore, John Hopkins University Press.

Ariès, P. (1981) *The Hour of Our Death*. Harmondsworth, Peregrine Books.

Blauner, R. (1966) Death and social structure. *Psychiatry*, **29**:378–94.

Cartwright, A. (1991) The role of residential and nursing homes in the last year of people's lives. *British Journal of Social Work*, **21**:627–45.

Counsel and Care (1995) *Last Rights*. London, Counsel and Care.

Field, T.M. and James, N. (1993) Where and how people die, in Clark, D. (ed.) *The Future of Palliative Care*. Buckingham, Open University Press, pp. 6–29.

Gorer, G. (1955) The pornography of death. *Encounter*, October: 49–52.

Hinton, J. (1972) *Dying*. Harmondsworth, Penguin.

Kearl, M.C. (1989) *Endings: A Sociology of Death and Dying*. Oxford, Oxford University Press.

Saunders, C. (1966) The last stages of life. *American Journal of Nursing*, **65**: 70–5.

Seale, C.F. (1995) Dying alone. *Sociology of Health and Illness*, **17**(3):376–92.

Shemmings, Y. (1996) *Death, Dying and Residential Care*. Aldershot, Gower Press.

Townsend, P. (1964) *The Last Refuge: A Survey of Residential Institutions and Homes for the Aged in England and Wales*. London, Routledge & Kegan Paul.

9 LONG-TERM CARE: IS THERE STILL A ROLE FOR NURSING?

Sally J. Redfern

The proposition of this book that a systemic understanding of care in communities requires a broader interpretation of 'institutions' is further developed in this chapter. So far, a variety of forms of institutional care have been discussed. In these chapters, the interdependence of formal and informal care, and of residential and community-based services, has been emphasised. The state, the family and numerous forms of residential and community care have all been identified as 'institutions' with a far greater degree of permeability than the conventional notion of the 'total institution' suggests. The nature and influence of professions as institutions has been touched upon in earlier chapters, and Professor Redfern's account of the changing nature and role of professional nursing focuses this aspect of the discussion. In doing so, this chapter offers further ways of addressing the urgent concerns of the previous two chapters about the effects of the rush to 'community care' on the quality of continuing care for the most vulnerable, sick and disabled people in our society.

The nursing press is full of talk about multiskilling clerical staff and porters to do the 'basic' nursing tasks, 'down-sizing' and 'rationalising' the nursing workforce, 'patient-focused care', 'hospital process engineering' and completely 'redesigning' health care delivery (see for example, *Nursing Times*, 22 February, 1995, p. 7; 1 March, 1995, p. 20). Nurses are worried. When a profession gets worried, it starts to examine what it is and what it does. This is what nurses are doing. The

NHS management argues that standards of care will not suffer from multiskilling the workforce. Rather, it says that much of the care currently carried out by nurses can be done just as well by support workers, thus freeing nurses to do the skilled nursing. This line of argument begs many questions, most notably the questions of what nursing is, where nursing is going and how the support worker's role can complement that of the nurse to meet patients' and residents' needs.

This chapter focuses on nursing care in institutional settings – residential homes, nursing homes and hospitals. It draws from nursing in the widest sense to explore what nursing is and where it is going. It looks at the multiskilling debate, including the wisdom of introducing a generic worker for care of elderly people and how best the support worker can complement the nurse's role.

First, some background. Even though there has been a major shift from long-stay hospital wards to smaller, local nursing home-type provision since the government White Paper *Caring for People* (Department of Health, 1989) and the National Health Service and Community Care Act 1990, the number of elderly people who live in residential or nursing homes has continued to grow (Tinker *et al.*, 1994). How many residential places are needed is not known, but what is known is the increasing level of stress on family carers who toil at home looking after old people who need continuing nursing care. There is no doubt that many of these old people need the services that only residential care can provide.

The policy to reduce the number of qualifed nurses and replace them with support workers, many of whom have had no training at all, has raised questions about the availability of people to give intensive and skilled nursing care. The government recognises the need for health and social services staff at all levels to receive training leading to professional, vocational or management qualifications, and expects all local authorities to develop and implement a training plan that takes the community reforms into account (Tinker *et al.*, 1994). Social services departments are encouraged to foster shared and joint training.

The NHS – through health authorities and fund-holding general practitioners – is responsible for arranging and funding services for people who require continuing health care. This includes continuing inpatient care in hospitals and nursing homes, and community health services for people in residential homes (Department of Health, 1995). The separation of 'health' from 'social' care does not serve the interests of people who need continuing nursing care. Skilled nursing straddles both and is not confined to high-tech nursing of the type needed in intensive care units and surgical wards. But what is skilled nursing?

What is nursing?

Nursing is under scrutiny more than ever before. Health service managers argue that many nursing tasks can be undertaken by support workers just as effectively, and more cheaply, as by nurses. In the face of this challenge, nurses are at pains to define the essence of nursing and its value to service users. Nursing journals are replete with articles that try to define nursing, but it 'seems to be now generally accepted in the realms of academic nursing that it is not clear what nursing is' (Bradshaw, 1995, p. 82).

Vaughan (1992) explores the kinds of knowledge needed for skilled nursing by giving examples of practice within Carper's (1978) four domains of 'knowing'. Nurses draw from medical and biological sciences for 'empirical or scientific knowledge' to understand why, for example, a person who has suffered a stroke misses one side of his face when shaving. His lack of awareness is the result of cerebral damage to the right hemisphere of the brain.

Nurses use 'personal knowledge of self' to understand, for example, why the urge to do things for the patient might override encouraging him to do it himself because the nurse will do a better job and do it more quickly. By understanding this personal knowledge domain, nurses check the urge and help the patient to shave the forgotten cheek and to understand why he had missed it.

'Aesthetic knowledge', which some observers refer to as 'artistry', involves the skills of 'being there' just at the time when a person needs a nurse. Benner (1984) calls this 'presencing'. For example, the skilled nurse knows 'without thinking' how to handle and help a person crippled with rheumatoid arthritis to move painlessly. The 'art' of nursing is based on tacit knowledge, intuition and reflection (Rose and Parker, 1994), which draw from Carper's personal and aesthetic knowledge. Skilled nurses can reflect on their actions whilst doing something else; they 'think on their feet', which requires the use of intuition and personal knowledge (Schön, 1983; Benner, 1984; Rew and Barrow, 1987). They use 'gut feelings' that rarely let them down about how to respond in a given situation without having to rely on rules, guidelines and procedures.

The fourth kind of knowledge is the 'moral knowledge which influences any act'. For example, the skilled nurse will intervene as an advocate if the surgeon plans to amputate an old lady's leg when she is determined not to have surgery and is well aware of the consequences.

Vaughan also reminds us of Habermas' (1972) three categories of knowledge: 'technical interest', 'practical interest' and 'emancipatory interest'. Technical interest refers to the nurse's technical and proce-dural competence that draws on theoretical knowledge. Practical interest is much more than getting the practical work done. It focuses on interpreting the meaning of nursing and the meaning of nurses' actions to patients. Others call this empathy (Baillie, 1995). Emancipa-tory interest refers to the power of critique, that is, the knowledge nurses need to act rationally, reason effectively and make decisions based on the available knowledge. Emancipatory knowledge promotes autonomy but, as Vaughan argues, is not well developed in nursing, although being essential for skilled practice.

The skilled and experienced nurse, referred to by Benner (1984) as an 'expert', acquires these types of knowledge through extensive prac-tice and continuing education and learning. All these kinds of knowl-edge are fundamental to skilled nursing in any setting, long-term hospital, nursing home and residential home included. They are not the province of health care assistants and other support workers, but support workers can learn to model themselves on knowledgeable nurses. This would ensure high-quality nursing care delivered by support workers under the supervision of nurses. It is unrealistic, and unnecessary, to staff all long-stay nursing settings only with nurses. But, if nursing no longer has a role within long-term residential care settings, the everyday fundamental nursing care that residents receive will not be skilled nursing care.

The nurse as an expert has been explored by Jasper (1994). She sees expertise as more than combining theory with practice and defines it as ' a specific mode of thinking which has evolved from the merger of knowledge, skill and experience' (p. 770). Experts can rely on heuris-tics, or 'rules of thumb', that allow them to bypass overt principles and the detailed steps of logical reasoning. This way of thinking – summed up as intuitive or tacit knowledge (Polanyi, 1967) and central to Benner's (1984) thesis – is not measurable but is, according to many opinion leaders, the crucial component that distinguishes the expert from the non-expert. Others, however, have criticised the over-reliance on intuition in attempts to define the expert nurse (English, 1993; Bradshaw, 1995).

Jasper's study with nurses on what 'expert' means puts more detail on her earlier definition. They saw an expert nurse as:

> a nurse who has developed the capacity for pattern recognition through high level knowledge and skill, and extensive experience in a specialist field, and who is identified as such by her peers. (Jasper, 1994, pp. 774–5)

Jasper (1994, p. 774) also identified antecedents and consequences of the expert:

Antecedents
1.   having confidence in oneself and one's decision-making skills;
2.   working with colleagues;
3.   exposure to a single environment within which skills and knowledge can develop; and
4.   holding appropriate basic qualifications in the chosen area and the opportuity to develop these.

Consequences
1.   accordance of high status within the profession;
2.   consultation by others; and
3.   use as a role model.

Caring in nursing

We have seen what kinds of knowledge underpin skilled nursing and what the expert nurse looks like, but a definition of nursing has not yet become clear. Nursing is often described as the major 'caring' profession, and 'care' is a common adjunct to nursing. It is as if 'nursing' is not sufficient to cover the whole domain subsumed within 'nursing care'. Some regard the term 'nursing care' as being tautological (Phillips, 1993), but an understanding of what caring is helps to clarify the nature of nursing.

The distinction between 'caring about' and 'caring for' or 'tending' a person is often made (Parker, 1981; Fealy, 1995). Caring about someone can range from mild concern to deep love, and caring for someone suggests provision for material needs such as shelter, food and security. Fealy adds 'looking after' as describing activities of a carer aimed at meeting individual needs, although the difference between caring for and looking after is not altogether clear. He also refers to some authors (for example, Downie and Telfer, 1980) who argue that caring does not require knowledge; rather, it requires a special kind of person who can communicate sensitively both verbally and non-verbally. Presumably, proponents of this view would deny the need for professional carers to possess different kinds of knowledge (scientific, personal, aesthetic and moral) and that health care assistants could be trained to take over the caring role from nurses. If this were the case, the nursing care of people living in long-stay institutional settings could become the responsibility of carefully selected health care assistants.

Caring is a complex phenomenon; it lacks clear definition and has been conceptualised in nursing in different ways (Watson and Lea, 1995). Watson and Lea explain that, at one end of the spectrum, caring is seen as unique *in* nursing (but not unique *to* nursing) and is the 'sole component of nursing' (Leininger, 1981; Watson, 1985). At the other end, caring is important but not unique in nursing (Benner and Wrubel, 1986). Others (for example, Phillips, 1993) argue that the focus on caring in nursing detracts from the concept of nursing and is not considered to be central to it.

Watson and Lea refer to Morse *et al.*'s (1991) five ways of conceiving caring:

- as a human trait (natural to being human);
- as a moral imperative (a fundamental human value);
- as an affect (extending oneself towards the person beyond what is necessary to do the job);
- as an interpersonal interaction;
- as a therapeutic intervention (deliberately planned with a predetermined goal).

The different theoretical perspectives on caring are succinctly distinguished by Watson and Lea. They describe three perspectives represented by Watson (1985), Leininger (1981) and Gaut (1983). Watson (1985) sees caring as unique in nursing and argues that it cannot be reduced to a series of tasks. Instead she defined caring as consisting of ten 'carative' factors, such as the development of a 'helping–trusting relationship', the systematic use of 'scientific problem-solving' to make decisions, assisting with 'gratification of human needs' and forming a 'humanistic–altruistic system of values'.

Leininger also regards caring as unique in nursing but believes that some aspects can be reduced to clearly defined activities. She distinguishes caring in a professional nursing sense from the generic caring that occurs when one person helps another. The professional nurse cares by using learned humanistic and scientific modes to enable people to improve or maintain their health. Thus professional caring, for Leininger, demands the kinds of knowledge mentioned earlier that go beyond the caring that any human being would give. Leininger developed a taxonomy of caring constructs that includes such aspects as 'comfort', 'tenderness' and 'touch', some, but not others, of which can be reduced to a measurable activity. According to Watson and Lea

(1995), Gaut believes that caring in nursing can be reduced to activities, and should be, so that it can be operationalised.

Research into caring in nursing tends to have taken a quantitative or a qualitative approach. Quantitative approaches into perceptions of the important dimensions of care show that nurses rate psychosocial skills, such as building trust and comforting people, highly, whereas patients rate the technical competence of nurses, such as monitoring the patient's condition and taking action if something is wrong, more highly (Kyle, 1995). Qualitative approaches, using a critical incident or repertory grid technique, have underplayed technical and physical tasks in nursing and have focused on how nurses act, for example their use of time and attitude towards patients, rather than on what they do (for example, Morrison and Burnard, 1991).

From their review of the literature, Watson and Lea list the following as caring dimensions in nursing:

- being supportive;
- empathy;
- competence;
- nurturing;
- involvement;
- attitude and liking;
- monitoring the patient;
- sensitivity;
- listening to the patient;
- approach to the patient and motivation;
- doing physical care;
- enabling and maintaining belief in the patient;
- explaining and facilitating.

They do not see this as a complete list, but it gives an idea of the range of dimensions that constitute caring in nursing. Few of these dimensions are themselves defined activities, but the activities within most of them could be defined and therefore be operational and measurable. It is, of course, the case that support workers carry out many activities within these dimensions, but they cannot work at the level of the skilled nurse. The patient would get short shrift if the support worker was left with responsibility for these dimensions. Watson and Lea argue that caring should be dissected to reveal its underlying dimensions so that the elements within each can be defined, understood and measured. Then they can be confirmed as therapeutic nursing interventions. From this preliminary work, they developed the Caring Dimension Inventory and found that four factors emerged as underpinning caring as perceived by nurses:

- psychosocial aspects of caring;
- technical and professional aspects of caring;
- personal disposition/altruism;
- involvement.

'Therapeutic' nursing care has become common parlance in the nursing literature, although what 'therapeutic' means is not always clear. Waterworth (1995, p. 13) defines it simply as 'care that makes a positive difference to patients'. She asked nurses to reflect on incidents when they had made a positive contribution to practice in a nurse–patient or nurse–relative encounter. From these, she identified broad categories of interventions that she aggregated into four dimensions that she described as nursing: a person-centred/person-focused dimension, an interpersonal dimension, a communication dimension and a team dimension.

To sum up so far, skilled, or expert, nurses have the capacity to recognise and react to patterns of activity displayed by a person whose health is compromised or potentially compromised. Nurses anticipate or respond to these behaviour patterns by applying different kinds of knowledge (scientific, personal, aesthetic and moral) to a range of caring activities. With these ideas in mind, we move on to consider where nursing is going and whether it will continue to keep responsibility for 'basic' nursing care.

Where is nursing going?

The kinds of knowledge and dimensions of caring described earlier are clearly important to nursing, but they could also be claimed by all the health professions, by social work and by other service professions, such as teaching. By arguing that dimensions like these can define what is unique about nursing, nursing is no further forward, important though they are. What seems to be missing from the earlier description of nursing is a declaration that nursing is fundamentally a set of practical activities around which relationships are built. The quality of the relationship determines whether the practical activity, and the relationship itself, is therapeutic. It seems to me that nursing has lost its focus on practical activities in its endeavour to demonstrate the distinction between skilled nursing care and doing a series of tasks in a mechanistic way. All nursing can be defined as a set of practical activities around which relationships are built, although the emphasis on relationships or technology varies according to the specialty; mental health nursing is more relational and intensive care nursing more technical, for example. In losing sight of practical activities as making up the essence of nursing, the uniqueness of nursing compared with the other 'caring' professions is unclear. This lack of clarity on what is unique about nursing could be its downfall.

We can see, then, that nursing is in danger of falling into the trap of which Aldridge, a social worker, warns us:

> The message from social work to nursing is thus: keep the technical skills in the foreground and build relationships upon them. It is not only more politically realistic but less destructively stressful. (Aldridge, 1994, p. 727)

Bradshaw, a nurse, drives a similar message home:

> nursing needs to recover a theory of nursing care that holds together the personal, the relational, the practical and the scientific and which helps nurses in partnership with all their colleagues to provide quality in care. (Bradshaw, 1995, p. 91)

She argues most forcibly that nursing academics in the UK have been totally confused by their struggle to find nursing's identity within the opposing and incompatible nursing theories that have winged their way from the USA. If the medical and physiological bases of care, common to the scientific, reductionist theories of Henderson (1966), Orem (1971) and Roy (1976), are abandoned or subordinated to the sociological, psychological and psychotherapeutic bases of care emphasised in the inductive interpretative theories of Reihl-Sisca (1989), King (1981) and Paterson and Zderad (1976), has this played into the hands of managers who want adequate care to be provided as cheaply as possible? Has the swing to the social sciences and away from the medical and biological sciences left nurses with no interest in body-care work, thus leaving them happy to give it away to untrained assistants? And, if nurses have given away fundamental body-care work, can they claim to provide holistic care?

Nursing, particularly the day-to-day 'basic nursing care', is under the microscope. There is universal agreement that basic nursing care belongs to nursing, but the question is who should do it? Managerial 'pragmatists' (Robinson, 1990), including health service managers, say that support workers are cheaper, better and preferred by patients (Brindle, 1993; Caines, 1993). Professional 'idealists' (Robinson, 1990), including advocates of the 'new nursing' and of the Project

2000/Diploma in Higher Education nursing education reforms, say that basic nursing care is fundamental to holistic, individualised nursing and needs professional qualified nurses if fragmented task-based care is to be avoided (Pembrey, 1984; Pearson, 1988; Salvage, 1990; Department of Health, 1991; Ersser and Tutton, 1991; Wright, 1991; Vaughan, 1995).

But nurses are expensive. They are expensive to educate, and they consume the largest proportion of the health services revenue budget. Like all professions in today's market-driven health service, nurses are under pressure to demonstrate their effectiveness and efficiency. Evidence for their effectiveness is, however, growing. Nurses have been shown to be directly associated with high-quality nursing care, and replacing them with untrained support workers is not the answer if standards are to be kept high:

> One of the recurrent findings in nursing is that the quality of patient care and outcomes are directly related to the quality of nursing labour, that is the educational preparation (Verran and Mark, 1992), nurses' grades (Carr-Hill et al., 1992) and the proportion of nurses in the workforce (Hancock, 1992). There have been data available in the UK since 1948 that the length of patient stay, as a proxy for state of health, is reduced and hence it is cost effective to have large numbers of nurses, rather than unqualified assistants... . (Bond, 1994, p. 2)

Advocates of the 'new nursing' movement, including government policy makers (Department of Health, 1989), argue passionately that 'primary nursing' is the way forward in the organisation of nursing work. Primary nursing stipulates that a primary nurse has responsibility, is accountable for and does all the nursing care for a small case-load of patients throughout their hospital stay, assisted by associate nurses who take over the planned care when the primary nurse is absent. The patient is included as a partner in the care process, and negotiation and liaison with other professionals is facilitated by the primary nurse rather than being fed upwards through the nursing hierarchy. This mode of working has been applied mostly to hospital nursing, but community nurses also follow its principles; many say that is the way they have always worked. In mental health care, key working is a close relation.

Effectiveness of primary nursing, compared with team and functional task-based nursing, has been claimed with respect to patient satisfaction (Bond et al., 1990), patient independence (Armitage et al., 1991) and cost (Thomas and Bond, 1991). However, other research has not found outcomes such as self-care management, patient well-being, stress and anxiety, life satisfaction, dependence, length of hospital stay and mortality to improve as a result of primary nursing (Thomas and Bond, 1991). Dewar (1992) carried out an activity analysis in a psychogeriatric ward that had changed to primary nursing. She found little difference in the quantity of direct care given by nurses compared with that by support workers, but the care differed in quality. Interpersonal communication by the nurses was greater and included provision of information and teaching, which the support workers did not do. The nurses could not, however, articulate their unique contribution to basic nursing care.

It is very difficult to define nursing outcomes when we are unable to describe clearly what nurses do that is uniquely nursing. Primary nursing is a good example of a mode of nursing intervention that has so far defied concise definition (Maguire *et al.*, 1994). If you cannot define it, you cannot measure its effectiveness. Bond's team is evaluating the effectiveness of the care of patients with fractured hip on outcomes such as level of pain, sleep, surgical complications and rate of gain in function and social activities on return home or to residential care (Bond, 1994). It is not clear whether or not the team will strive to disentangle aspects of the care process that are uniquely nursing. They may argue that it does not matter who is responsible for the inputs as long as the outcomes for the patient can be measured.

Pure primary nursing, in which all nursing care is delivered by nurses, is unrealistic in long-stay residential settings and is also unnecessary. Practice partnerships, in which the primary nurse works in direct care assisted by support workers, is more effective than team nursing or task-oriented nursing, in which nurses and support workers also work together (Thomas and Bond, 1991). That is, there are significant differences between modes of working but not between the quality of nurses' and support workers' care within modes. Thomas and Bond found that, compared with team nursing and task-based wards, the nurses in primary nursing wards did more basic nursing care, engaged more in therapeutic discussion with other professional colleagues, and more often gave patients choice, explained the planned care to them and asked them questions to discover their wants, to assess their needs and to seek their agreement to the care planned.

Paid non-professional helpers come in many guises – as auxiliaries, support workers, health care assistants, housekeepers and clerks. I have tended to refer to them collectively as support workers, but two different roles have been identified: the enabling role (clerical work and housekeeping) and the assisting role (those who give direct care supervised by the nurse). Other supporter roles are 'care technicians' (with specialised functions in X-ray departments and renal units, for example), nursing aides, who have some autonomy and discretion in decision making, and 'generic helpers' who assist a range of professionals. The nurse acts as teacher, adviser, supervisor and controller (Dewar and Macleod Clark, 1992).

The literature points to nurses' mixed feelings about the advent of a large body of support workers. Negative reactions focus on fear of losing their role and concerns about slipping standards. Positive reactions include relief that help is on hand to take over non-nursing work so that they can get on with direct nursing (Dewar and Macleod Clark, 1992). The evidence available, although pretty meagre, suggests that, when nurses and support workers work in a complementary way through a personalised partnership, as in primary nursing, the quality of nursing is high and the workforce is happy. A way of working that weakens the boundary between what nurses do and what support workers do, yet ensures that nurses keep control, responsibility and accountability for nursing work, has clear benefits for cost-effective care.

The effectiveness of nurses and health care assistants working in community hospitals and units for people with learning disabilities has been evaluated by Ahmed and Kitson (1993). They found that, although primary nursing was in operation, the lack of a coherent framework for the organisation of care left ambiguity and confusion among the staff. In the community hospitals, the primary nurses were the direct care-givers and the associate nurses supported them, but, when the primary nurse was absent, the consistency and continuity of care broke down. The auxiliaries gave very little direct care. In the learning disability units, health care assistants gave all the direct care and were out of their depth with clients whose needs constantly changed. The 'primary nurses' were remote from direct care and concentrated on developing a 'team leadership' role. It is clear that assistants' roles in each setting need careful definition. Assistants need the support of a primary nurse who is involved in a sufficient amount of direct care to be a role model and who takes a close and continuing supervisory role.

We can conclude that evidence for the effectiveness of primary nursing in enhancing quality of nursing care is growing, but we still do not know exactly what the process is that leads to better nursing. Tierney (1992) has made a start in defining nursing inputs, which could be related to patient outcomes but which vary from being distinct and distinguishable as nursing to being indistinct and indistinguishable (Figure 9.1). If nurses from all specialties revised and expanded the inputs in Figure 9.1 to fit their area of work, outcomes associated with nursing itself and nursing as a contribution to health care more widely could be defined.

Distinct	Discrete nursing interventions (e.g. mouth care)	Distinguishable
	Composite nursing interventions (e.g. bowel management)	
	Total nursing care (i.e. individualised, holistic nursing)	
	Systems of nursing (e.g. primary nursing, key working)	
	Dedicated nursing services (e.g. community psychiatric nursing)	
	Nursing input to multiprofessional health care (e.g. reminiscence therapy, sexual awareness counselling)	
Indistinct	Nursing input to health care plus other inputs (e.g. discharge planning)	Indistinguishable

Figure 9.1 *Nursing inputs (after Tierney, 1992)*

This section has considered where nursing may be going in meeting the challenges it faces, particularly how it can preserve personalised care within a broadened skill mix configuration. I have described what is emerging as a definition of nursing and what are outcomes of nursing care. A fundamental question is whether nursing will continue to own basic nursing care even though nurses may have help from support workers in providing it.

Will nursing keep basic nursing care?

It could be said that nurses who have not moved to primary nursing have the advantage if the goals of the market reforms in today's health service oppose and prevent the individualism and holism advocated by the 'new nursing'. How does this market approach square with the continuing urging by the Department of Health Nursing Division (Department of Health, 1993) to nurses to adopt individualised patient care, holism and the 'named nurse' approach?

The power of the market reforms suggests that nursing is moving back to task-based practice so that health care assistants can keep the 'production line' going with nurses as shop floor supervisors. Although nursing representatives close to government continue explicitly to endorse the value of the 'new nursing' to the quality of nursing practice and the professionalising of nursing, there seems to be an implicit move back to task-based practice within the ethos of 'patient-focused care', 'standard clinical protocols' and 'care pathways' (Luker, 1995).

However, if we accept Pearson's (1988) assertion that basic nursing care is a skilled and important activity, it cannot be delivered if health service managers give it only lip service or if it is added on as an extra to be done when nurses are not tied up with being 'technicians, skivvies, handmaidens or clerical officers' (Johns, 1994, p. 157). There has to be a way of resolving the chasm between professional concerns that embrace nursing care and organisational structures that are concerned about efficient management and cost reduction. Johns is amongst many opinion leaders who are concerned about nurses' roles being extended to take on some of the junior doctor's technical tasks so that their hours can be reduced without reduction in their work. Trust managers, Johns tells us, assume that nurses can take on this work with no extra resources. Something has to give, and it is likely that this will be direct care activities that give skilled nurses the opportunity to do so much more than the physical task:

> Direct care activities such as bathing will be delegated even more to untrained staff – and yet it is these opportunities that nurses tell me are the opportunities to 'know' their patients. (Johns, 1994, p. 158)

This extension of nursing into medical care is as relevant to nursing care in residential settings as it is to acute hospital and community care. The opportunity for nurses to 'know' the residents, using the scientific, personal, aesthetic and moral ways of knowing described earlier, will be lost. Intermittent supervisory visits by nurses to support and monitor support workers' work are not sufficient for this kind of relationship to develop. The outcome will be to deny residents access to therapeutic basic nursing care.

The generic worker?

Does the supervisor of support workers doing the basic nursing care in long-stay residential care settings for elderly people have to be a nurse? Could it be another health care professional? After all, many newly qualified nurses reject a career in long-stay hospital and nursing home settings because it is too 'basic' and 'wastes' their training. They seek the rewards of the 'medical model', with its emphasis on, preferably, cure, but rehabilitation if cure is out of reach.

The medical model is clearly not appropriate for the long-term care of elderly residents, but Nolan (1994) argues that nurses who advocate a nursing model for care of elderly people (for example, Kitson, 1991) are equally misguided if, as is widely accepted, one of the fundamental concepts underpinning care of old people is multiprofessional team work. Nolan's view is that discipline-specific models of care contradict the notion of holistic care that the 'new nursing' espouses; fragmented care must surely result. He argues that the search for a 'geriatric nursing model' runs the danger of being 'professionally reductionist' within an agenda of 'professional protectionism'. He illustrates clearly the conflict between the need for an holistic and integrated health care knowledge base for the care of older people and the desire for professionals to increase their own specialist knowledge base to enhance their power and prestige.

Along with Nolan, we can see the attractions in Hollingberry's (1993) call for 'a new trans-disciplinary profession' for meeting many of the care needs older people require. Hollingberry argues that a properly educated and qualified generic worker – the 'gerocomist' – would meet the needs of older people much more effectively than the fragmented care they get, or should get, today. As Nolan reminds us, 'gerocomy is derived from "old age tending" as opposed to geriatric (old age) treatment' (Nolan, 1994, p. 994), so is more appropriate for most old people. The core knowledge and skills that would be shared across professions would have to be identified, and this would be the responsibility of the gerocomist. All students wishing to work with older people would be educated together. They would all qualify as gerocomists and some would specialise by taking further training.

This suggestion of a generic worker will be regarded as heresy, Nolan admits, by many professionals, particularly those, such as nurses, who are only just beginning to define their knowledge base. However, from the service user's point of view, a generic worker with a basic knowledge of nursing, medicine, physiotherapy, occupational therapy, clinical psychology and social work as applied to gerontology and the care of older people is likely to meet all their care needs. More specialist knowledge will be needed by the few. In the meantime, given that Hollingberry's suggestion is too radical for both established and fledgling disciplines to contemplate, an increase in the opportunities for shared learning will encourage much more effective interprofessional working than the lip service given to multidisciplinary team working that commonly occurs at present.

The proliferation of 'nursing development units' (Salvage and Wright, 1995) has done much to raise the profile of nursing and to provide a basis from which a knowledge base for nursing can develop. However, as nursing matures as a discipline, its territorialism (professional protectionism) may decline, thus allowing the single-discipline nursing development units to advance into multiprofessional 'practice development units' (Williams *et al.*, 1993).

Practice development units, and nursing develoment units, have a great potential for continuing care of all kinds – for young physically disabled people, old people, people with learning disabilities and people with mental illness. They can be based in any kind of residential setting – hospital, nursing home, residential home, hostel. For old people the generic worker with a wide repertoire of skills and knowledge from the health and social work professions could be the answer. As Nolan (1994, p. 995) says, 'nursing is a vital ingredient in the health and social care mixture' and, if it has the confidence to shed its 'mantle of protectionism and reductionism', it could make a profound contribution to improving the care of older people of all ages and in all settings, including continuing residential care.

Conclusion

Nurses have always worked with support workers, so the introduction of health care assistants and other helpers is controversial, not so much because nurses fear being displaced by support workers, but because they are under pressure to define what nursing is (Wynne, 1995). If they do not, someone else will, and, if that happens, the indefinable essence of what skilled nursing is will be lost. Nursing will be reduced to a series of tasks that health care assistants, trained to a specified level of competence, could do.

Is there still a role for long-term residential care institutions, and, if so, is there still a role for nursing in them? Given that the proportion of very old people relative to the younger elderly age group is rising, many will continue to need extensive and continuing nursing care. There has to be provision of good quality 24-hour-a-day, 7-days a week nursing in institutional settings as well as in people's homes if the stresses for family carers are to be lifted. If professional nurses disappear entirely from institutional settings, the loser will be the resident, who will be denied the therapeutic basic nursing care that the possession of scientific, personal, aesthetic and moral knowledge bring. But a partnership between the skilled nurse and support worker can preserve the essence of therapeutic nursing and high-quality care. Transforming the skilled nurse into a professional gerocomist could be an attractive proposition for the care of elderly people. It would enhance continuity of care and would avoid the fragmentation common to present-day professional inputs. It would also increase the professional standing of nurses and other health care professionals who choose to work with elderly people.

References

Ahmed, L.B. and Kitson, A. (1993) Complementary roles of nurse and health-care assistant. *Journal of Clinical Nursing*, **2**:287–97.

Aldridge, M. (1994) Unlimited liability? Emotional labour in nursing and social work. *Journal of Advanced Nursing*, **20**:722–8.

Armitage, P., Champney-Smith, J. and Andrews, K. (1991) Primary nursing and the role of the nurse preceptor in changing long-term mental health care. *Journal of Advanced Nursing*, **16**:413–22.

Baillie, L. (1995) Empathy in the nurse–patient relationship. *Nursing Standard*, **9**(20):29–32.

Benner, P. (1984) *From Novice to Expert*. Menlo Park, CA, Addison-Wesley.

Benner, P. and Wrubel, J. (1986) *The Primacy of Caring*. Menlo Park CA, Addison-Wesley.

Bond, S. (1994) What Are Outcomes of Nursing Care? Paper presented at the Passport to Quality Conference, London, 22–24 June.

Bond, S., Fall, M., Thomas, L. and Bond, J. (1990) Primary Nursing and Primary Medical Care: A Comparative Study in Community Hospitals. Report 39. Newcastle Upon Tyne, Univeristy of Newcastle, Health Care Research Unit.

Bradshaw, A. (1995) What are nurses doing to patients? A review of nursing theories past and present. *Journal of Clinical Nursing*, **4**:81–92.

Brindle, D. (1993) Measuring the quality of care. *Guardian*, 16 June:15.

Caines, E. (1993) Amputation is crucial to the patient's health. *Guardian*, 11 May:20.

Carper, B. (1978) Fundamental patterns of knowing in nursing. *Advances in Nursing Sciences*, **1**(1):13–23.

Carr-Hill, R., Dixon, P., Griffiths, M. *et al.* (1992) *Skill Mix and the Effectiveness of Nursing Care*. York, University of York, Centre for Health Economics.

Cassidy, J. (1995) *Nursing Times*, 22 February: 7.

Department of Health (1989) *A Strategy for Nursing*. London, Department of Health Nursing Division.

Department of Health (1991) *The Patient's Charter*. London, HMSO.

Department of Health (1993) *A Vision for the Future*. London, NHSME.

Department of Health (1995) *NHS Responsibilities for Meeting Continuing Health Care Needs*, HSG (95) 8, LAC (95) 5. London, Department of Health.

Dewar, B-J. (1992) Skill muddle? *Nursing Times*, **88**(33):24–7.

Dewar, B-J. and Macleod Clark, J. (1992) The role of the paid non-professional nursing helper: a literature review. *Journal of Advanced Nursing*, **17**:113–20.

Downie, R.S. and Telfer, E. (1980) *Caring and Curing: A Philosophy of Medicine and Social Work*. London, Methuen.

English, I. (1993) Intuition as a function of the expert nurse: a critique of Benner's novice to expert model. *Journal of Advanced Nursing*, **18**:387–93.

Ersser, S. and Tutton, E. (eds) (1991) *Primary Nursing in Perspective*. Harrow, Scutari Press.

Fealy, G. (1995) Professional caring: the moral dimension. *Journal of Advanced Nursing*, **22**:1135–40.

Gaut, D.A. (1983) Development of a theoretically adequate description of caring. *Western Journal of Nursing Research*, **5**(4):313–24.

Habermas, J. (1972) *Knowledge and Human Interest*. London, Heinemann.

Hancock, C. (1992) *Nurses and Skill Mix: What are The Issues?* London, Royal College of Nursing.

Henderson, V. (1966) *The Nature of Nursing*. London, Collier Macmillan.

Hollingberry, R. (1993) *Gerocomist: A New Trans-disciplinary Profession*. Paper presented to the British Society of Gerontology Conference, Norwich, September.

Jasper, M.A. (1994) Expert: a discussion of the implications of the concept as used in nursing. *Journal of Advanced Nursing*, **20**:769–76.

Johns, C. (1994) Can human caring in practice be an everyday reality for nurses? *Journal of Nursing Management*, **2**:157–9.

King, I. (1981) *A Theory of Nursing*. New York, John Wiley & Sons.

Kitson, A. (1991) *Therapeutic Nursing and the Hospitalized Elderly*. London, Scutari Press.

Kyle, T.V. (1995) The concept of caring: a review of the literature. *Journal of Advanced Nursing*, **21**: 506–14.

Leininger, M.M. (1981) The phenomenon of caring: importance, research questions and theoretical considerations, in Leininger, M.M. (ed.) *Caring: An Essential Human Need*. Thorofare, New Jersey, Slack, pp. 3–16.

Luker, K. (1995) Research and the configuration of nursing studies. Winifred Raphael Memorial Lecture, November, London, Royal College of Nursing.

MacGuire, J., Adair, E. and Botting, D. (1994) *Primary Nursing in Elderly Care*. London, King's Fund Centre.

Morrison, P. and Burnard, P. (1991) *Caring and Communication: The Interpersonal Relationship in Nursing*. London, Macmillan.

Morse, J.M., Bottorff, J., Neander, W. and Solberg, S. (1991) Comparative analysis of conceptualisations and theories of caring. *IMAGE: Journal of Nursing Scholarship*, **23**(2):119–27.

Nolan, M. (1994) Geriatric nursing: an idea whose time has gone? A polemic. *Journal of Advanced Nursing*, **20**:989–96.

Orem, D. (1971) *Nursing: Concepts of Practice*. New York, McGraw-Hill.

Parker, R. (1981) Tending and social policy, in Goldberg, E.M. and Hatch, S. (eds) *A New Look at the Personal Social Services*. Discussion paper number 4. London, Policy Studies Institute, pp. 17–32.

Paterson, J. and Zderad, L. (1976) *Humanistic Nursing*. New York, John Wiley & Sons.

Payne, D. (1995) *Nursing Times*, 1 March: 20.

Pearson, A. (1988) Trends in clinical nursing, in Pearson, A. (ed.) *Primary Nursing: Nursing in the Burford and Oxford Nursing Development Units*. London, Croom Helm, pp. 1–22.

Pembrey, S. (1984) Nursing care: professional progress. *Journal of Advanced Nursing,* **9**:539–47.

Phillips, P. (1993) A deconstuction of caring. *Journal of Advanced Nursing,* **18**:1554–8.

Polanyi, M. (1967) *The Tacit Dimension.* New York, Doubleday Anchor.

Reihl-Sisca, J. (1989) The Reihl interaction model: an update, in Reihl-Sisca, J. (ed.) *Conceptual Models for Nursing Practice,* 3rd edn. Norwalk,CT, Appleton & Lange, pp. 383–403.

Rew, L. and Barrow, E.M. (1987) Intuition: a neglected hallmark of nursing knowledge. *Advances in Nursing Sciences,* **10**(1):49–62.

Robinson, J. (1990) The role of the support worker in the health care team. *Nursing Times,* **86**(37):61–3.

Rose, P. and Parker, D. (1994) Nursing: an integration of art and science within the experience of the practitioner. *Journal of Advanced Nursing,* **20**:1004–10.

Roy, C. (1976) *Introduction to Nursing: Adaptation Nursing.* New Jersey, Prentice Hall.

Salvage, J. (1990) The theory and practice of the 'new' nursing. *Nursing Times,* **86**(4):42-5.

Salvage, J. and Wright, S. (1995) *Nursing Development Units: A Force for Change.* Harrow, Scutari Press.

Schön, D.A. (1983) *The Reflective Practitioner.* London, Maurice Temple Smith.

Thomas, L.H. and Bond, S. (1991) Outcomes of nursing care: the case of primary nursing. *International Journal of Nursing Studies,* **28**(4):291–314.

Tierney, A.J. (1992) Outcomes that reflect nursing input, in Bond, S. (ed.) *Outcomes of Nursing: Proceedings of an Invitational Developmental Workshop.* Newcastle upon Tyne, University of Newcastle, Centre for Health Services Research, pp. 28–32.

Tinker, A., McCreadie, C., Wright, F. and Salvage, A. (1994) *The Care of Frail Elderly People in the United Kingdom.* London, HMSO.

Vaughan, B. (1992) Exploring the knowledge of nursing practice. *Journal of Clinical Nursing,* **1**:161–6.

Vaughan, B. (1995) Celebrating 25 years of primary nursing. *Journal of Clinical Nursing* Editorial, **4**:69–70.

Verran, J.A. and Mark, B. (1992) Contextual factors influencing patient outcomes, individual/group/environment interactions and clinical practice interface, in *Patient Outcomes Research: Examining the Effectiveness of Nursing Practice,* Proceedings of a conference sponsored by the National Center for Nursing Research, US Department of Health and Human Services.

Waterworth, S. (1995) Exploring the value of clinical nursing practice: the practitioner's perspective. *Journal of Advanced Nursing,* **22**:13–17.

Watson, J. (1985) *Nursing: Human Science and Human Care. A Theory of Nursing.* Norwalk, CT, Appleton-Century-Crofts.

Watson, R. and Lea, A. (1995) *A Postal Survey and Multivariate Analysis of Perceptions of Caring Among Nurses Working in Lothian.* Edinburgh, University of Edinburgh, Health Department of Nursing Studies.

Williams, C., Lee, D. and Lowry, M. (1993) Practice development units: the next step. *Nursing Standard,* **8**(11):25–9.

Wright, S. (1991) Of primary importance. *Nursing Times,* **87**(10):38–41.

Wynne, T. (1995) Skill-mix in nursing: efficiency and quality? *Journal of Nursing Management,* **3**:189–91

10 When and How Institutions Do Work – The Caring in Homes Initiative

Leonie Kellaher

This chapter begins by briefly revisiting the conventional critique of the total institution and, as in previous chapters, pointing to its inadequacies in terms of an analysis of the potential of today's residential institutions to play a part in enabling communities to care. The previous chapter addressed the issue of what constitutes quality in continuing care from the perspective of the nursing profession. Leonie Kellaher now turns our attention to the structures of residential institutions and how these can facilitate quality care. Throughout this book, the preservation of individual identity in the face of physical or psychological dependency has been a recurrent theme. Institutions of all types that intervene to provide care – formal and informal, residential and community based – may threaten this identity. Practice-based research over the past 30 years has shown us ways in which the aspiration to preserve the self within the institution can be attained.

A great deal of research has been undertaken over the past three or four decades which attempts to explain institutional life: what it is, why it takes the shape it does, and what those who experience it think and feel. Much of this research has focused on the workings of institutional establishments for older people, the numerically largest group living in residential settings. The analysis offered in this chapter springs from research experience and observations made in these settings by the

Centre for Environmental Studies in Ageing (CESSA), where earlier research findings on residential settings, particularly for older people, have generated the argument that a built environment supporting the individual is likely to be both a precondition for and an indicator of proper social and emotional support (Willcocks *et al.*, 1987). A more recent review (Peace *et al.*, in press) of the last decade's research and policy concerning residential homes for older people has extended this argument to assert that recognition and support for the essential self of residents is essential if the institution is to be judged successful in terms of recent policy statements and of the aspirations of a generation with new expectations. It follows that institutional practice and custom that make difficult the lifelong impulse to determine the self and maintain identity must be regarded as falling short of the ideal – if not the norm.

Whilst research and policy in relation to residential homes for older people form the basis of discussion and arguments put forward in this chapter, it is clear that those who live and work in institutions, or residential homes – the currently preferred nomenclature – have characteristics in common, despite differences in age, in physical fitness and in mental frailty. The Caring in Homes initiative, a major programme of research and development, considered residential care across the board, covering all the main care groups; the evaluators found:

> that the common needs and interests of those living in residential homes outweigh the differences. (Youll and McCourt-Perring, 1993, p. 3)

The term 'residential institution' is used in this chapter since it is held that 'institution' need not continue to carry pejorative connotations. Nonetheless, one of the aspects of living in residential settings, whether the resident is a child of 8 or 9, or an older person in their eighties or nineties – perhaps with cognitive impairment – a younger person with physical disability or someone recovering from drug or alcohol misuse, is that, sooner or later, he or she will run up against the institutional buffers. In other words, freedoms will be restricted as the interests of the collectivity come to prevail over those of the individual. This is, of course, not the only instance in which individual inclinations become subordinate to those of a collectivity. The family and other groupings in society also restrict individual intention and agency. The institution, however, restricts in particular ways and often with consequences that have come increasingly to be regarded as undesirable, both for individuals themselves and for the community or society.

Institutions, in the broadest sense, are arrangements that have their legitimacy in the society that engenders them and permits them to function. They encompass people in what are judged, by that community or society, to be appropriate groupings, to attain certain goals, which are also sanctioned by society. This does not by any means imply that those grouped together and bounded by institutions always have the same characteristics. To observe the family as an institution is to see that the idea of 'institution' is not synonymous with internal homogeneity. In the case of the family, of educational settings and so on, the institution is arranged in such a way that internal diversity can be accommodated, and the potential for individual development follows. The problem with closed or total institutions, such as many residential settings, is that the resident group being supported or treated within the institutional boundary loses diversity and individuals become institutionalised (Goffman, 1961). In writing about the idea and reality of 'institution', Foucault has taken the most tightly bounded of society's institutions, prison, as an exemplar of society's restrictive and repressive facets (Foucault, 1967). Whilst Goffman's observations and analysis have dealt with everyday life, as well as life in very restricting settings, he has also tended to focus upon those aspects of living, in both bounded and open settings, which tend to limit, if not maim, the self, the personality. The individuals whom Foucault and Goffman have considered are rendered similar, within the boundaries of establishments, by strategies such as block treatment. It can be argued that these influential writers have taken a telescopic view that focuses very sharply on the closedness of institutions in society, rather than the view that locates the institution in a broader, more diffuse context and permits exploration of permeability in the boundaries that distinguish institution from community.

This is not to say that such observations of institutions as repressive instruments of society are inaccurate. There are many data supporting the analysis of institutions as restrictive and, sometimes, cruel places. Townsend's descriptions and analyses (Townsend, 1962) translate Foucault's and Goffman's propositions in terms of familial institutions, notably the old people's home, which are located close to, if not in, their communities. It may now be possible to make the case, in the mid-1990s, that institutions can be perceived as less monolithic and in different relationship with community or society than may have been the case until the last decade or so. In other words, that, as the philosophies underpinning the recent legislation work through, the residential settings that have previously been depicted as closed and institutionalising could become more open and located somewhere along the continuum of care which the community should offer to those who need support from time to time.

The meaning of the label 'residential' was hammered out in the early 1980s, for a range of client groups, with the drafting and enactment of the Registered Homes Act 1984. Those establishments to be registered and regulated under this Act were ones which provided varying permutations of accommodation, board and care of a personal – although not necessarily physical – nature for groups of individuals who had particular sets of needs for support. This could be for support over very long, continuous or fragmented periods, or for brief periods of time. It was significant that establishments providing for four or fewer people remained outside the jurisdiction of the Registered Homes Act until its amendment in 1992, the message being carried that board and personal care might be delivered at the institutional or domestic level and that the latter was to be outside regulatory range. In the event, the apparently domestic frequently turned out to be institutional in a different, commercial, sense rather than in terms of block treatment being meted out to three or four people.

It has to be acknowledged that institutional settings, for the full range of client groups, have undergone significant transformations over the past decade or so. The large mental hospitals have 'decanted' their patients into small group living homes. Children's homes have been subject to unprecedented examination. Residential and nursing homes for older people are now generally smaller-scale operations than those which characterised the period before the Registered Homes Act 1984. Personal space has been increased, with reductions in the numbers who must share rooms with non-kin, and enhanced with more private toilet and bathroom provision. It is also, however, necessary to ask whether institutions – residential homes – may, despite appearances, be essentially the same, limiting settings because the internal structures, and those which connect the establishment with its community and society as a whole, remain unchanged.

In this chapter, ideas on what may characterise or engender institutions that are more or less successful will be considered. The possibility of institutional transformation is raised, with the proposition that new structuring principles must be applied to the long-recognised elements that constitute the residential institution. Ways in which this might be wrought are considered, with emphasis on quality assurance in residential care, and Inside Quality Assurance (IQA) (Kellaher, 1995) as just one approach. A new institutional culture is tentatively proposed as an incipient reality indicating that a valid sense of self need no longer be a threat to potential residents if certain structures and dispositions are in place.

Successful and unsuccessful institutions

The research tradition in which residential settings for older people are concerned has generally been to examine the data collected about residents, staff, the regime and the physical environment, and to arrive at analyses concluding that the lives of residents lack autonomy and often the dignity that accompanies a sense of agency. This is variously attributed to residential structures – buildings, staff training, poor links with the community – that disempower all concerned, and to societal structures that legitimate and buttress these residential lapses (Baldwin *et al.*, 1993). Sometimes, the capacities of the frail resident are cited as an explanation for the lack of autonomy frequently taken as an indicator that something is not working properly. Suggestions for improved practice may follow, but the inference to be drawn from the research of the 1960s, 70s and 80s is that, whilst there are frequent instances of good practice, these generally occur at the individual rather than institutional level, depending upon the skill of particular members of staff and special staff–resident relationships. This may be more typical of old people's homes than establishments for other groups, such as children, where resident staff ratios are more balanced and the proportion of staff with appropriate training is likely to be higher. Thus the research findings produced through academic work and the Social Services Inspectorate point to structural lapses and offer explanation and remedy.

Policy statements – more or less informed by research – have invariably urged that individuals must be respected. These statements have also, generally, framed residential living in a positive and optimistic light. The Wagner report (Sinclair, 1988) and the code of practice *A Better Home Life* (Centre for Policy on Ageing, 1996) have elaborated the principles of good practice. The importance of dignity and respect are stressed, as are basic rights as citizens, along with proper scope for self-determination and individuality and the desirability of living a full and active life (Centre for Policy on Ageing, 1996, p. 7). The schemes, such as *Homes Are for Living In* (Department of Health/Social Services Inspectorate, 1989) for assessing how far these principles are present in a home, and how they are lived out, similarly stress values such as dignity, fulfilment, choice and so on.

Despite the analyses of residential settings to have emerged from research and policy statements, it is not easy to form a picture of what a successfully working institution would look like on the ground. Residents are to be treated respectfully and their aspirations and capacities for autonomous action are to be encouraged. It is possible, as already suggested, to cite instances in which individual residents have these good experiences. Institutional structures supporting such good practice are, as a matter of course, less frequently described as the norm. It is arguable, however, that institutions only 'work' when they do so at the structural level. The 'charismatic' approach, founded on the inspired manager, the devoted staff members and close individual relationships, cannot be a substitute for structure since it at best engenders uncertainty, and at worst exposes all concerned to the organisational capriciousness that can only induce dependency.

The residential institutional elements of buildings, organisation and resident characteristics have been referred to. What is proposed here is that these 'ingredients' can be juxtaposed structurally or randomly. In the latter case, the institution may operate successfully for some of those involved, but it is undoubtedly vulnerable to failure as an institution. Where there is a sound structural foundation, the institution is less at risk. Whether it is successful or unsuccessful is a judgement dependent on criteria which, as already noted and as will be further considered, have been subject to shifts over time. It is obvious that, in certain – perhaps organisational – respects, the residential institutions which Townsend described were successful; but they were not successful in terms of resident well-being. It may be argued that the character of a residential institution is determined by the way in which the essential components are arranged. In the following section, two structuring principles are put forward.

Different sets of interests

The observation that different sets of interests are entailed in creating and maintaining residential institutions is not a new one. Indeed, it underpinned the work of Foucault, Goffman and Townsend, but it is a fact that has been obscured by the overgrowth of domestic and familial analogy to have accumulated around residential care. Images of home, of family and of domesticity have obfuscated the real nature of residential institutional living for decades. The frequent refrains 'It is just like their home here' and 'We don't have rules, you don't have rules at home' have served to confuse staff and residents alike, and to undermine the benefits to be derived from shared living in certain circumstances.

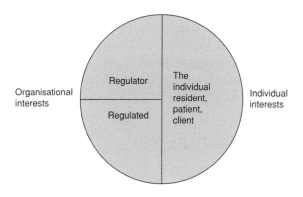

Figure 10.1 *Different sets of interests*

The fact is that, in residential institutions, however small, there are distinct sets of interests (Figure 10.1). On the one hand, staff have a working life to maintain; they have interests around conditions of employment, remuneration and the way in which work impinges on their personal world. The owner or manager has similar interests but is additionally concerned with the establishment's image and reputation, as with its future prosperity in financial and moral terms. The residents are concerned to be as comfortable, secure and content as they can be in a shared setting. Above all, they must preserve their sense of self. It is arguable that much of the institutional behaviour observed in residential settings for old people – watching the television, defending territory (chairs and dining room places) and keeping a distance and not joining in – are devices for preserving the self in settings where it may be threatened. Relatives and friends have sets of interests that are only partly aligned with those of residents. Like staff, relatives and friends have lives elsewhere, which must be conducted in parallel to the residential life. Those responsible for regulating the character and standard of institutional life, similarly, have different sets of interests which, nonetheless, impinge on residential life.

The recognition of the different sets of interests noted above must be the basic structuring principle if residential institution is to work successfully, which in this context means to the benefit of the resident group for whom it is established. Without such a recognition, strong organisational influences will always overwhelm the influence that can be exerted by residents who are not only individuals, but also vulnerable in other ways. Unless there is clarity of where resident interests are delineated, these cannot be properly defended. Regulatory activity – registration and inspection – is based upon the requirement of offseting strong organisational influence and supporting the weaker individual. Internal regulatory activity will need to follow a parallel path. Both perspectives should permit a balancing of individual and organisational interests. This balancing represents the second structuring principle.

Balancing individual and collective

The setting of a balance between the weight of the organisation and that of the individuals who live and work in a setting is crucial in determining how particular residential settings work and in whose interests they function. It is, as noted above, a relationship that underpins all regulatory activity. Residential institutions have their *raison d'être* in their residents. If the institution is to be judged minimally acceptable, it must arrange itself in such a way that the individual can be recognised and supported within the collectivity of shared living arrangements. This balance, which is implied in residential arrangements and in the range of regulatory activity that includes inspection, registration and contracting, is illustrated in Figure 10.2. The traditional residential elements are included, but equal prominence is given to the day-to-day events that constitute the experience of living and working in a residential institution. This second structuring principle allows a balancing act that takes account of resident interests alongside those of other parties. In turn, the way in which influences and interests are balanced will yield the prevailing residential institutional climate.

The components of residential institutional life shown in Figure 10.2 – building, organisation and resident mix – have frequently been employed as frames and bases for research and policy development. Regulatory and, more recently, contracting activity rest upon consideration of these categories and assessments of the standards that are reached for each of them. It is arguable, however, that institutions only work, in the sense of serving the interests of residents, when these elements are articulated in certain ways to produce the properly balanced background climate. Furthermore, the institution works when this climate is such that it allows individuals good chances to be themselves in an environment where living and organisation must be based on principles of sharing and economies of scale and which are not domestic or familial. If the institutional climate produced, through the recognition of discrete sets of interests and the balancing – or regulation – of organisational and individual interests, does not support the individual, it may, in terms of criteria now elucidated in legislation, policy documents and codes of practice, be said not to work.

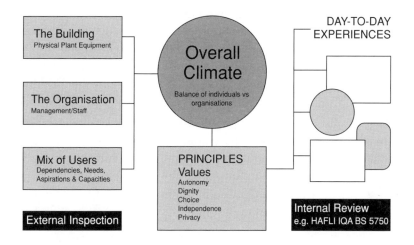

Figure 10.2 *Balancing interests and creating a residential/institutional climate*

The achievement, and then the maintenance, of such a balanced climate is clearly a delicate and difficult process. It may still be the case that few residential institutions have managed to reach this point of balance, but the thrust of effort since the enactment of the 1990 Community Care and Health legislation has been to find ways and develop systems that make attainable institutional environments with the capacity to support and reconcile individual and collective concerns.

Institutional transformation

Work in residential institutions in the 1990s has been characterised by attempts to link the realities of everyday residential experience with the categories and rhetoric put forward as desirable in the research recommendations and policy statements of earlier decades. At least in part, this is a consequence of refinements in regulatory procedures, which increasingly take account of the resident viewpoint on outcomes and the requirements of the contract culture in which minutiae of the residential experience are examined as these are produced and delivered.

The Wagner report *A Positive Choice*, which reviewed research findings and policy statements on residential life for all groups of people, made a number of recommendations for action to transform the residential option from a residual to a positive one, alongside options for care and continued support in the domestic setting. This report, and subsequent Department of Health initiatives (Department of Health/Social Services Inspectorate, 1989), represents one example of efforts to build better institutional structures by moving from rhetoric and pronouncement to an emphasis on developmental action, on the residential ground.

A Positive Choice listed ten recommendations for ensuring that the nature of residential provision would be transformed in such a way that it would be regarded by the community at large and by potential residents as a desirable option when extra support became necessary. Four of these were identified as important, and the Caring in Homes initiative was set up in 1989 to develop schemes for introducing and continually reinforcing each of the four recommendations in the full range of residential establishments covered by the Registered Homes Act 1984 and in less traditional settings such as refuges. The development of a system for internal review of the residential institution was one of the four strands of the Caring in Homes initiative. The production of IQA was the outcome to the developmental work undertaken by CESSA. The IQA system for internal review of the range of residential settings was based upon earlier research on the interrelationship between the three residential elements (Peace *et al.*, 1982) and on the two structuring principles outlined above.

The point here, of discussing how IQA was developed, is to illustrate how the workings of residential institutions – the attainment of a good balance of interests and a beneficial climate – can be influenced in the day-to-day experiences and responses of residents and others concerned: in other words, how institutional transformation might take place so that new criteria replace longer-standing ones in weighing up whether a residential institution does or does not work.

IQA: one approach to changing culture

The development of IQA started from an assumption that there would always be a need for some residential accommodation for each of the client groups for whom provision had traditionally been made. It also took as a starting point the view that, despite all the research findings, the CESSA's included, to have emerged up to and particularly during the 1980s change in residential settings, certainly for older people, whilst to some degree evident in the physical environment, did not appear to have been either fundamental or radical in organisational terms. A radical approach was to be adopted. This acknowledged that the resident, however unwilling or unable to give voice an observation, should be regarded as the central and most valuable source of information on how the institution was working and how it might work better.

The idea that 'insiders' are the best people to report on the minutiae of day-to-day living in the relatively closed settings that are many residential homes – for all groups and not just older people – requires some expansion, if not defence. As a general rule, the research and thinking on residential provision (for example, Davies and Knapp, 1981; Booth, 1985) has assumed that the most permanent institutional elements are those of physical environment and organisation. The point that the resident group, in terms of its particular requirements rather than as individuals, is the most consistent element of residential living tends to have been overlooked by both researchers and practitioners. Observing, as they necessarily do, from outside, they fail to notice that neither physical fabric nor the organisation remains constant, even for the duration of an individual resident's stay in care. There are changes often to buildings and constantly to staffing arrangements.

The belief that any information from insiders is better than no information formed the basis of an approach that did not insist on random or statistical 'sampling' to provide a starting point for new understandings of residential institutions. So in developing IQA, the rationale for placing the resident centrally was this: that it was not only fair, but also logical, to regard the resident – or the residents' collectivity – as the most fixed element. It followed that the accounts given by this group of their residential experiences had to be given great weight, something which was beginning to be voiced as an ideal in 1990 but not quite taken seriously in terms of actions.

The mechanics of IQA, as a quality assurance system for use within institutional settings, are described elsewhere (for example, Kellaher, 1992, 1995; Kellaher and Veitch, 1993). Here it is sufficient to outline the main supports that steer the process.

1. IQA is a step-by-step process leading to an account of the institution, its work and its aspirations, as expressed by those within – residents and staff – although others connected with the institution may also be involved.
2. The IQA process, which takes time, sometimes 2 or 3 months, is steered by a group made up of both insiders and outsiders.

3. Informants are guided to comment on their experiences of the residential institution by considering a small number of very general topics. They are prompted to describe their experience and then to say how things might be different: description and diagnosis.
4. The information collected from a range of constituencies of different sets of interests already noted is weighed up. Dominant themes are highlighted for consideration and action as appropriate over time.
5. The intention is that the IQA exercise be undertaken on an ongoing basis every year or so.

This summary of IQA, as a system that has been developed through a series of trial demonstrations involving up to 200 residential institutions for all groups of people across the sectors, illustrates just one way of refocusing concerns about residential living through the comments of those who experience and receive services day by day, rather than through those who organise. Importantly, in terms of the argument being put forward here, IQA is:

• a framework for opening up the institution – to itself in the first instance; in this respect, it takes account of the structural principal that a range of discrete sets of interests be acknowledged;
• a system that permits the different, and sometimes opposed, views of the various parties to be fairly reviewed and balanced against each other;
• a strategy for legitimising the voice of comment, and sometimes criticism, from residents and others;
• the systemisation of ordinary comment on day-to-day experience.

The mechanics and principles underpinning IQA are, as noted above, intended to capitalise on the insider's expertise in evaluating how a residential institution is working at a particular time, and to check imbalances, as well as to enhance the climate so that individuals have a good chance to be themselves in a shared setting. Can it do this? Can a system such as IQA bring about the institutional transformation required if an institution is to be evaluated as working well in the light of the criteria that the new legislation has heralded?

New institutional cultures?

It seems clear that, over the past decade, residential institutions have changed their appearance and that, in some areas, standards have been raised. It is rare now, for example, for older people to be in multi-sharing rooms. Such shifts, visible in the physical environmental aspects of institutional care, do not, however, in themselves change the nature of care, although they are preconditions for and indicators of change for other aspects that are less easily charted.

In their evaluation of the impact of IQA, within the Caring in Homes initiative as a whole, Youll and McCourt-Perring (1993, p. 51) cited a number of benefits accruing to residents, and to others concerned. First, they suggested, 'The direct impact on the residents themselves in being involved' was possibly the most significant outcome of an in-house review involving insiders as experts, in that levels of expectations might be shifted: 'Even where residents did not say much or speak freely, it seemed that the experience opened up possibilities for the future.' In several homes, 'Residents gained confidence both in their ability to speak out and in the results of doing so.' One resident complained about a member of staff well after the review had ended. It appeared that she had taken time to consider whether it was worth complaining and had then chosen when and to whom she would talk (Youll and McCourt-Perring, 1993, p. 52).

Second, Youll and McCourt-Perring reported the impact that the IQA review had on the material environment and the running of the institution itself. Third was the impact on the attitudes and practices of staff and others, such as outside professionals, relatives and local people. The evaluation team suggested that the benefits to residents were strongly associated with the manner in which the review had been carried out. Where resident involvement was minimal, impact tended to be relatively small scale.

One of the indicators that the institutional climate might have been adjusted through the opening-up process that IQA aims to bring about is that the chances of residents being themselves are raised. Three comments from managers suggest that this can be, or might become, the case:

> Once residents' confidence in the IQA system has been developed, I feel that it should enhance their chances.
>
> I think IQA will make it possible, but it is only the beginning of a long process.
>
> It is likely to make possible as it provides a safe setting for people to state their views and feelings.

An analysis of the way in which residents express their ideas through a process such as IQA, in which a degree of openness and attributability is combined with a measure of anonymity, is given in 'Rest assured' (Kellaher and Peace, 1993). Ten points were identified that hint at ways in which a new openness in institutional residential settings may become manifest:

- Users say quite a lot when asked to respond in their own terms.
- People make observations about the day-to-day detail of institutional life rather than about structural issues. Resident comment sometimes concerns matters of such detail that outsiders, may dismiss it as imperceptible or even insignificant.
- Residents of all groups are well able to focus their remarks on the service being provided, on the routines and the way things appear to be organised.
- People make suggestions for change which are practicable and generally with reasonable resource implications.
- People say things repeatedly, though in different forms, it is relatively easy to pick out half a dozen or so timely themes which concern informants.
- Residents do not say many things which surprise the other groups of informants, though staff may be jolted at first by the power of a collectivised resident voice on a limited number of issues.
- Occasionally there may be a hint that all is not well and something needs airing or further exploration.
- Residents make comments rather than criticisms.
- They balance criticism with appreciation.
- They hint rather than make direct remarks.

There is, then, the possibility that the institutional culture, in establishments for older people at least, may be amenable to change, which leads to nearly imperceptible shifts – which is not to say that they are unimportant – in resident willingness to open up in expressing views and ideas. Increasingly, residential institutions, using a range of quality assurance and control schemes, are attempting to open up their still ill-understood and closed worlds, both to themselves and to outsiders. Some of the quality strategies involve residents, as do regulatory mechanisms, although not all place residents centrally as informants. Change in physical and material environments has also been observed, and, in these respects, residential institutions are now more comfortable and possibly more private than hitherto.

A crucial question remains, however, of how far any observed trans-formations, even if only in a small proportion of residential institu-tions, are fundamental or cosmetic. It is too early to pronounce on the permanence of beneficial changes reflecting the adoption of the two structuring principles considered in the earlier part of this chapter. It is possible, however, that the responses of older people to residential care may provide a litmus paper on the nature of recent transformations. Critically, is the residential option one which older people now plan for and choose with a lighter heart?

In some instances, for some individuals, the move to residential care may be motivated by a willingness to opt for the supports of residential living (Willcocks *et al.*, 1987). It has to be said, however, that for a majority of older people – and those who fall into other residential groups – continued struggle against admission is more usual. In other words, institutional care continues to be set apart. One of the influ-ences on older people that leads to resistance, even though residential institution is now likely to appear welcoming, is the enormous effort that residents of all ages and with a range of particular care require-ments still have to make in order to maintain a sense of self in the insti-tutional setting. How is this wariness, beyond the guardedness that might reasonably be expected of people unconnected by kinship or history, to be explained? Residents still make remarks such as, 'I didn't think it would come to this!' What is it in residential institutions that remains so threatening where the explicit care is the goal? One response is that the threat to self is so serious that older people have only capitulated in the past after considerable erosion of will has taken place, and they may then live to regret the chink in their defences. It is not the move from home that threatens. Older people move into shel-tered housing, which may entail as much contact with care providers as would be the case in the residential setting. They may do so, with regret at leaving a home they have known for decades, but the sense of defeat that can accompany a move to residential institution is not char-acteristic of the move to special housing.

Conclusion

This chapter is about the circumstances in which institutions may work, in the new sense of working for the residents, which, of course, entails functioning well as an organisation. Whilst attention has been given to the possibility that residents and potential residents remain anxious that their sense of self and identity is at risk in the residential institution, a case has been made that this is not now always so, and that old ideas about institutionalisation may now be less appropriate. Furthermore, an argument has been proposed that the elements constituting the residential institution need no longer rest on structuring principles that permit only a crude articulation which cannot accommodate, and much less resolve, the tension between individual, collective and organisational interests.

Of course, new principles for structuring and shaping residential institutions may be ignored, as they entail an engagement with residents, staff and others that is not traditional and is not an easy option. Such engagement will both require and engender greater openness about the institution. It is only in such circumstances, however, that residents will, in the longer term, accept that they have a real and active part to play in the ongoing task of shaping the institutional environment. Only if this re-patterning takes a firm hold, on a wider scale, will residential institutions lose their threat for resident groups. Youll and McCourt-Perring, writing on IQA, make a point that goes beyond this particular scheme:

> What the IQA system sets in place is not a series of standards or definitions of quality but the people and constituencies of interest who are able to debate, define and implement these in relation to a particular home. (Youll and McCourt-Perring, 1993, p. 61)

Such an approach is more likely than others that are concerned with elements as static entities to support the development of an institution that reveals diversity. This diversity, the antithesis of the block treatment characterising institutions that can no longer claim to 'work', may appear in a number of dimensions: in appearance, of the place itself, but especially of the residents; in mood, at different times; in expression and communication; in activity; and in disposition to the past, present and future.

Diversity can only emerge if the individual is secure in an institutional climate that is appropriately balanced. Balance will be possible where there is sufficient knowledge of the different sets of interests and where those involved have the confidence, as well as willingness, to regulate the influences, so that even the weakest and most vulnerable individual is not overwhelmed by strong collective and organisational forces. At root is the maintenance of self. A residential institution cannot be judged as working if it cannot arrange itself so that residents, potential residents and those who care for them are secure in the certainty that the self will not be eroded and undermined. There is modest but accumulating evidence that institutional transformation is becoming possible and that residential provision can become a positive option.

References

Baldwin, N., Harris, J. and Kelly, D. (1993) Institutionalism: why blame the institution? *Ageing and Society*, **13**(1):69–82.

Booth, T. (1985) *Home Truths: Old People and the Outcome of Care*. Aldershot, Gower.

Centre for Policy on Ageing (1996) *A Better Home Life: A Code of Good Practice for Residential and Nursing Home Care*, Report of an Advisory Group convened by the Centre for Policy on Ageing and chaired by Kina, Lady Avebury. London, Centre for Policy of Ageing.

Davies B. and Knapp M. (1981) *Old People's Homes and the Production of Welfare*. London, Routledge & Kegan Paul.

Department of Health/Social Services Inspectorate (1989) *Homes Are for Living In*. London, HMSO.

Foucault, M. (1967) *Madness and Civilization*. London, Routledge.

Goffman, E. (1961) *Asylums: Essays on the Social Situation of Mental Patients and Other Inmates*. New York, Anchor Books.

Kellaher, L. (1992) *IQA: Inside Quality Assurance, The IQA Action Pack*. London, Centre of Environmental and Social Studies in Ageing and Information Design Unit.

Kellaher, L. (1995) IQA: Inside Quality Assurance – its rationale and use in residential and non-residential settings, in Pilling, D. and Watson, G. (eds) *Evaluating Quality Services for Disabled People*. London, Jessica Kingsley, pp. 164–79.

Kellaher, L. and Peace, S. (1993) Rest assured: new moves in quality assurance for residential care, in Johnson, J. and Slater, R. (eds) *Ageing and Later Life*. London, Open University and Sage, pp. 168–77.

Kellaher, L. and Veitch, M. (1993) The Inside Quality Assurance Programme, in Leiper, R. and Field, V. (eds) *Counting for Something in Mental Health Services*. Aldershot, Avebury Press, pp. 53–60.

National Institute for Social Work (1993) *Positive Answers: Final Report of the Wagner Development Group*. London, HMSO.

Peace, S., Kellaher, L. and Willcocks, D. (1982) *A Balanced Life: A Consumer Study in a Hundred Local Authority Old People's Homes*. London, PNL Press.

Peace, S., Kellaher, L. and Willcocks, D. (in press) *Re-evaluating Residential Care*. Buckingham, Open University Press.

Sinclair, I. (1988) *Residential Care: The Research Reviewed*. London, HMSO.

Townsend, P. (1962) *The Last Refuge*. London, Longman.

Wagner, G. (1988) *Residential Care: A Positive Choice*. London, National Institute for Social Work.

Willcocks, D., Peace, S. and Kellaher, L. (1987) *Private Lives in Public Places*. London, Tavistock/Routledge.

Youll, P.J. and McCourt-Perring, C. (1993) *Raising Voices: Ensuring Quality in Residential Care: An Evaluation of the Caring in Homes Initiative*. London, Brunel University/HMSO.

11 WHY AND WHEN INSTITUTIONS DO NOT WORK – *SANS EVERYTHING* REVISITED

Mervyn Eastman

The focus of the previous chapter on the structural reasons for the failure of residential institutions leading to the neglect of personal identity and how they can be realistically mitigated addressed the abuse of selfhood. In this chapter, Mervyn Eastman draws on the literature of dysfunction – the litany of residential care failure – to identify what the managers of residential institutions can and should be doing to minimise the risk of all forms of abuse. As he points out, the facts of abuse within residential care have been disclosed regularly over 30 years – what is puzzling is why such abuse still occurs despite the acknowledged changes in residential institutions over this period. This chapter suggests that, whilst there has been an undeniable catalogue of abuse in residential care, its roots lie not in the nature of residential institutions as such but in the much larger 'institutions' – institutionalised ageism in society and the power structure of welfare organisations – within which they exist and are managed.

Blockages – their causes and effects

It was 1967 when Thomas Nelson published Barbara Robb's indictment of the frightening conditions endured by older people in some hospitals and nursing homes – *Sans Everything* (Robb, 1967). As a young social worker, I read Robb's disturbing account with total disbelief. I had not, either as a student or a social work practitioner, encountered such abuses in homes that I visited nor heard from my managers that they were dealing with such practice. It was not until some years later that, in the role of manager, I found myself having to confront practice that could only be understood in the context of abuse in residential care.

Toileting a resident with the bathroom door wide open; shouting at residents or ordering them around; intimidation; ignoring; inflexible routines; refusing residents a meal; poorly made beds; over/under-medication; lack of stimulation – all these remain in the 1990s the experience of too many people in the care of local authority and independent homes. There is no need to prove that such behaviour is abusive or that it is still being perpetrated in many homes today, but the question remains, 'Why'? More specifically, how is it that the individual managers of residential care homes and their line managers at all levels either actively engage in such practice or collude with its existence? When staff or residents disclose abuse, why does the organisation insist on 'evidence beyond reasonable doubt' rather than on the balance of probabilities'? Why insist on a second witness? Why deny that the abuse can possibly happen in one of our own homes?

The answer probably lies between total management incompetence and blatant collusion, whereby the individual resident is marginalised or discounted. The key message is that managers who fail to recognise or, even if disclosed, fail to confront abuse are more culpable than is the member of staff who has physically or emotionally abused the resident. The sadistic punishments meted out to children in residential care justified crudely as a behavioural therapeutic regime ('Pindown') did not happen in secret: they were practised openly for any senior manager who cared to read the daily log book or listen to the child. Nye Bevan Lodge did not happen overnight but over a long period of time, culminating in the 1987 enquiry revealing a lengthy history of continual abuse of every kind perpetrated on elderly residents. Abuse therefore occurs, it occurs regularly and is there to see. What are the blockages that prevent directors and their management teams, proprietors or trust boards seeking out abuse and confronting it in their residential homes?

This chapter focuses primarily on older people given that community care spending on this client group far exceeds that on others; however, the issues arising are equally applicable to any client group. I suggest that there are four key blockages, or blind spots, that may help to account for this managerial ineffectiveness leading to the continued abuse of vulnerable people:

- *Ageism* – negative stereotypes of and attitudes towards older people.
- *Ignorance* – unawareness of what constitutes abuse in residential homes and not knowing what to look for in a home that 'appears to be running well'.
- *Denial* – a mindset denying that abuse is occurring.
- *Fear* – avoidance of confrontation.

Ageism, ignorance, denial or fear are the cornerstones on which residential abuse has for decades been based.

Ageism

It is assumed that senior managers – who are still drawn from the rank and file of professional practice – have a positive attitude towards ageing and therefore older people. However, Kayser-Jones found that the most frequently reported complaints against staff were infantilisation, depersonalisation and dehumanisation (Kayser-Jones, 1992). How are these attitudes related to the inaction of managers in the face of abuse? First, in treating older people as difficult, challenging, irresponsible or undependable, managers view a disclosure of abuse as unreliable given the 'victim's' age, mental health status and contributing behaviour.

Second, the regime of the home structurally re-inforces through the block treatment of people who are not regarded as individuals with personal preferences. Raymond Jack pointed to the way in which the policy of homes closures or transfers into the independent sector involves the social work profession in what he calls 'institutionalised abuse' (Jack, 1992). The wishes of residents not to close their home or not to be transferred are simply overridden by a policy of 'enforced relocation'. Such a policy to close a home without adequate regard to the wishes or needs of individual residents is an example of what Kayser-Jones call depersonalisation.

Finally, if those views are not even requested or are ignored in the decision making process, how can managerial decision making take into account the capacity of residents to assume responsibility for their own lives? If it does not, this constitutes a form of ageist dehumanisation.

Ignorance

Unawareness of what constitutes abuse or not knowing what to look for is commonplace. Experts in the field of elder abuse continue to debate what it is, and, given this uncertainty it is hardly surprising that practice agencies find it hard to define. Nevertheless, given that definitions of and guidance on policy and practice do exist – for example, the Social Services Inspectorate Policy Guidance *No Longer Afraid* (Social Services Inspectorate, 1993a) – it is difficult to understand how so many agencies caring for older people continue to operate without such policy and practice guidelines. Managers, when asked in the Social Services Inspectorate study *Confronting Elder Abuse* (Social Services Inspectorate, 1993b) what they considered the difficulties associated with recognising abuse (albeit in this case in the domestic setting) were, highlighted the following problems:

- reluctance of the abused person to disclose;
- establishing that abuse was occurring;
- fabrication of disclosure;
- the belief that physical abuse is harder to define than financial abuse.

Despite this research base – including an exhaustive study of the numerous abuse scandals in residential homes for older people by Clough (1992) – which could offer guidance, most staff are still in ignorance as very few agencies have guidelines that specifically identify what constitutes abuse. Consequently, managers do not know what to look for in terms of the factors that predispose the abuse of residents. It is as if the visiting manager, failing to personally witness a resident being abused, believes that such abuse is non-existent.

Drawing on this research, I would propose the following factors as relevant indicators:

- The power balance within the home.
- Staff factions often based on conflicting positions over so-called traditional or progressive regimes.
- High staff turnover.
- Low staff morale.
- Domestic appliances or furnishings that are in need of repair or replacement.
- Inspection reports.
- A number of apparently minor incidents that establish a pattern.
- Staff uncertainty over the aims and objectives of the home.
- Too few or too many complaints.

Denial

A powerful piece of work undertaken by Julia Wardhaugh and Paul Wilding, coining the phrase the 'corruption of care', examined where caring services or institutions go wrong. They point out that managers either failed to take action in spite of countless complaints or 'turned a blind eye' to what goes on providing the home continued to function in an outwardly acceptable fashion (Wardhaugh and Wilding, 1993). The reasons for such responses are numerous, but in my view they all have in common a lack of personal vision by the managers. In other words, they have lost sight of the individual older person's dignity, and, without a powerful conviction of the individual worth of each resident, they fail to recognise their individual responsibility to preserve it. Symptoms of this lack of vision and conviction are statements such as:

- 'It's not my responsibility.'
- 'Nobody can tell me what I don't know.'
- 'I can't allow staff to tell me what to do.'
- 'I have to keep complaints contained "in-house".'
- 'I'm too busy.'
- 'It's not as bad as all that... .'
- 'There's no policy or practice guidelines to tell me what to do... .'
- 'It will reflect badly on me and harm the home's/department's reputation.'

Wardhaugh and Wilding emphasise that what is significant about the 'corruption of care' is the totality of management failure. It is my assertion that the totality is not surprising if homes managers are themselves managed by visionless managers who have lost sight of their primary managerial task and obligation – to meet the needs of vulnerable people with dignity and respect.

Fear of confrontation

Over the past 30 years, much has been written on abuse in residential institutions, which refers to the fear both residents and staff have in disclosing abusive practice: fear of being isolated, blamed, disloyal, being sacked. Little attention has, however, been paid to the fear of middle, senior or executive managers. In understanding this blockage, one needs to examine the organisational culture that exists. Holman (1993) has argued that the so-called 'New Right' belief in and promotion of market forces and competition has led to selfishness and greed, and that the contract culture in health and welfare has brought a realignment of social work from a 'caring profession' to a cut and thrust buying and selling business. The corollary of this is that organisations reward macho-management, tough decision makers and keeping costs down. Those managers who hold onto the values of the 1960s and 70s are perceived as 'past their sell-by date'. I disagree. Personal advancement and ruthless ambition have always existed in the statutory welfare services, but the, admittedly destructive, stagnation of a 'job for life' in the 1960s has given way to employment insecurity of the 1990s. The fear of being made redundant, being seen as ineffective in resource management and being 'politically incorrect' has fostered a culture that is non-confrontational. Thus managers who fail to own personal responsibility will place the blame elsewhere and/or be afraid to take risks when abuse is eventually disclosed.

Users and their carers are often fearful that a complaint will lead to a denial or withdrawal of a service. It is my contention that staff who are devalued by their managers will be unable to sustain regard for their client. A culture that reinforces blame will be a culture of fear, non-confrontation and managerial sycophancy. Managers who feel under siege, have negative attitudes about their organisation, their department or themselves and the future cannot sustain an approach to those residents in their care that focuses on high-quality responses or 'human standards' in service provision. Non-confrontation is also occasioned by the fear that 'I may by wrong.' There is a good deal of ineffective confrontation: that which does not bring about change or improvement in staff performance. If there is one skill woefully absent in the management of residential care, it is the ability to confront effectively.

Confronting the blockages

Having examined the four blockages of ageism, ignorance, denial and fear, what is to be done to ensure that managers take responsibility, confront their own limitations of knowledge and expertise, and break down the barriers that lead to abuse in residential care?

Creating positive images of ageing

Managers throughout the organisation should continually reflect on their perception of old age. Chris Phillipson and Simon Biggs have produced an excellent section in their training manual *Understanding Elder Abuse* regarding ageism and the experience of abuse (Phillipson and Biggs, 1992). They identify a number of tasks that, if undertaken, could assist care staff in dealing with negative stereotypes of older people; these tasks are easily adapted for the manager:

- Examine any problems within our own relationships with ageing relatives, particularly if they are becoming dependent.
- Explore difficulties in communication across generations. Do we relate differently to older workers?
- Recognise our individual fears about the process of ageing.
- Be aware of our own ageist attitudes and those of our organisation and society.

As the authors point out, challenging ageism must be central to any strategy aimed at tackling abuse and neglect. Any manager who fails to challenge his or her own ageism will be ill equipped to confront the conditions in the workplace. Simply producing policy and practice guidelines is not enough.

What constitutes elder abuse?

Agreeing an agency definition of abuse is crucial. The London Borough of Enfield has reviewed regularly its own definition agreed by elected members, which is as follows:

> The physical, emotional or psychological abuse of a vulnerable adult by a formal or informal carer. The abuse is repeated and is a violation of an individual's civil human rights by a person or persons who have power over the life of a dependant.

This definition attempts to include abuse in residential care and is supported by a section in the authority's practice guidelines (London Borough of Enfield, 1993) specifying what constitutes abuse. Other definitions, such as that used by Bennett and Kingston (1993), prefer the terms 'mistreatment' or 'inadequate care'. Whatever the definition, the agency needs to make clear the moral judgement it is making. Staff operating in residential care are ill served if their managers do not make clear what is unacceptable practice.

Identifying the predisposing factors

Having examined previously those factors managers frequently ignore, agencies may find it helpful to draw together a matrix of indicators based on the works of Clough (1992), Phillipson and Biggs (1992), Wardhaugh and Wilding (1993), and Eastman (1984). The ability of visiting managers to 'see, hear and taste' the symptoms whilst walking around the home, speaking with residents and staff, is crucial. Additionally, the manager will only be able to identify those factors if the blockages previously discussed above are unblocked.

Abuse happens in my homes

When I originally researched elder abuse in a domestic setting (Eastman, 1984), I was confronted by the notion that I could be a potential victim and/or abuser. Likewise, managers need to address the same uncomfortable issue. Nye Bevan Lodge may well have been a home run by a local authority, but the lessons remain applicable to any care agency. Southwark have to be congratulated for openly establishing the original enquiry in 1986; other authorities might have kept their own 'dirty linen' private.

Let us remind ourselves of some of those lessons:

- All care agencies must look closely at what is happening in their own establishments.
- Staff who behave uncaringly or insensitively should be confronted and – if their behaviour is abusive – removed.
- Responsibility rests with the senior management team.
- Each home should have clearly written aims and objectives supported by an admission and complaints procedure that is monitored.
- Staff training needs to be identified and acted upon, including setting up an appraisal system.
- A code of practice should be developed which all staff are required to sign.

Furthermore, it should be emphasised that any manager who becomes aware of deterioration in a home's standards should act to resolve the problem. In the context of community care initiatives, Phillipson and Biggs produced what has turned out to be a useful checklist, worthy of consideration by homes' managers:

- Methods of restraint and control evaluated.
- The physical environment of the home examined for its effect on the morale of residents and – I would add – staff.
- A regular evaluation of residents who are socially isolated.
- How far residents are encouraged to participate in various activities.
- Staffing ratios that allow for the maximum stimulation of residents.
- Elder abuse training.
- Policy and guidelines on abuse.
- Quality circles.
- Advocacy.
- The level of contact with relatives.
- Quality control and assurance with published performance indicators.

Whilst emphasising the need for policy and practice guidelines, it should be stressed that, without adequate monitoring of their use and therefore effectiveness, they are in themselves meaningless.

Confrontation of fear

Managers who control, centralise decision making and bully are the most managerially insecure. Their personal fear of being seen to be ineffective leads to inefficiency and the continuation of abuse.

What therefore are the qualities of effective homes managers?

- They are self-confident, with a positive self-image.
- They perceive each and every resident and staff member as having inherent worth and dignity.
- They understand the purpose and function of residential care in the context of the organisation in which it is located.
- They are well organised and plan their work priorities.
- They are good at both written and verbal communication.
- They are flexible.
- They confront poor practice, both professional and managerial, of their own staff, peers and line managers.
- They are aware of their blockages.
- They are supportive and praise/reward disclosure.
- They have the ability to apologise.

- They are comfortable in seeking advice and owning up to what they do not know.
- They vary their style of leadership and delegate effectively.
- They involve staff in decision making.

(Adapted from Wagner, 1991.)

Demonstrating these qualities will assist the central managerial task of confrontation, in particular the confrontation of abuse in residential care.

Lessons for effective confrontation

If abuse is occurring or suspected, what can the manager do having first owned responsibility for it?

- Be clear about why confrontation is necessary – to change abusive practice and/or behaviour.
- Articulate very clearly what behaviour is unacceptable and why.
- Confrontation is more effectively undertaken on a face-to-face level rather than by letter, memo, telephone call or staff meeting.
- Contract to confront, for example 'I am concerned about some things you are doing/not doing. Are you ready to hear them at this time?' This requires clear management decision making.
- Confrontation is more successful if the staff member's dignity and self-respect is left intact. Very few people are inherently 'bad' – what is required is to confront the abusive behaviour.
- Determine whether the confrontation requires a light touch.
- Listen to residents when they complain or disclose and let them know you understand and what action you are going to take.
- If you are angry, express anger at the time you are likely to be heard.
- Always be in control (rather than controlling) and self-confident.

(Adapted from Wagner, 1991.)

In the event that none of these approaches is effective, it may be necessary to increase the scale of confrontation, but, depending on the nature of the abuse, confrontation may need to culminate in a report to the police and/or formal disciplinary action. Many managers are reluctant to move into this necessary stage of confrontation; the decision is often seen to rest elsewhere in the organisation. Many abuses have continued because managers not directly involved in the care of the older people hold the ultimate decision on whether to progress disciplinary action; it is therefore important that their blockages are confronted.

Sans everything

One is tempted to conclude that, over the past 30 years, little has changed in residential care, especially that of older people. Such a conclusion would be unjustified; certainly, my own experience of over 25 years is that much has improved. Nonetheless, despite improvements such as in the design of buildings, improved quality assurance and complaints procedures and so on, abuses still exist and are there for anybody with an eye to see, an ear to hear and, by no means least, a heart to care. Management today, as it did yesterday, has a case to answer. Using Robb's Shakespearean quote, we too often continue to be without teeth, eyes and taste – in fact, sans everything.

References

Bennett, G. and Kingston, P. (1993) *Elder Abuse: Concepts, Theories and Interventions*. London, Chapman & Hall.

Clough, R. (1992) Scandals in residential centres: a report for the Wagner committee, in Phillipson, C. and Biggs, S. *Understanding Elder Abuse: A Training Manual for Helping Professionals*. London, Longman, p. 115.

Eastman, M. (1984) *Old Age Abuse*. London, Age Concern.

Holman, B. (1993) *A New Deal for Social Welfare*. Oxford, Lion Books.

Jack, R. (1992) *Institutional Abuse*. BASELINE No. 50. Newcastle Under Lyme, British Association of Services for Elderly People, pp. 24–7.

Kayser-Jones, R. (1992) in Phillipson, C. and Biggs, S. (eds) *Understanding Elder Abuse: A Training Manual for Helping Professionals*. London, Longman. p. 3.

London Borough of Enfield (1993) *Abuse of Vulnerable Adults Guidelines*. London, Enfield Social Services Departments.

Phillipson, C. and Biggs, S. (1992) *Understanding Elder Abuse: A Training Manual for Helping Professionals*. London, Longman.

Robb, B. (1967) *Sans Everything*. London, Thomas Nelson.

Social Services Inspectorate (1993a) *No Longer Afraid*. London, HMSO.

Social Services Inspectorate (1993b) *Confronting Elder Abuse*. London, HMSO.

Wagner, A. (1991) *The Transactional Manager. How to Solve People Problems with Transactional Analysis!* Denver, T.A. Communications.

Wardhaugh, J. and Wilding, P. (1993) Towards an explanation of the corruption of care. *Critical Social Policy*, **13**(37)1.

12 THE FUTURE OF RESIDENTIAL CARE – A PERSONAL VIEW

Richard Clough

In this concluding chapter, Richard Clough, in his personal view of residential provision since the Second World War, draws together the concern shared by all the previous authors about the depletion of public residential care facilities for the most disadvantaged groups in our communities, the ill-informed basis on which it has been justified and the obvious inadequacy for so many of 'community care'. The existence of, and potential for more, high-quality residential care integrated within its community is described and the urgent need for a greater confidence in this form of social care provision – and in those who provide it – is powerfully reaffirmed.

Residential care has become an issue for consideration perhaps as never before. The public have had residential care brought to their attention as changes in provision, funding and practice have brought major anxieties to a public that previously cared little about a service that has simply 'been there'. Institutions have never, in the UK, been seen as part of the community. This attitude was partly caused by placing institutions at the edge of town or in the former country houses of the 'great and the good'.

Public awareness of residential care has increased for several reasons. The fact that people now live longer and are likely to become more infirm with increasing age means that the chances of being able to cope in their own home have lessened. In 1995 there were well over half a million people in the UK who were elderly, chronically ill or physically disabled living in registered homes or hospitals. By far the largest percentage in occupancy were elderly people, who in England and Wales accounted for 260,000 places. With these figures, the chances of a relative being in a registered home have considerably increased.

Issues relating to funding of residential care have meant that an inheriting society was under threat as people were forced to sell property that they would have formerly passed on to relatives in order to pay for care in their final years. In the face of these developments, service users and relatives have taken the opportunity to have a much greater say in what sort of service they expect to receive, and quality assurance and standard setting have become essential elements in the increasingly competitive 'business' of residential care – just as in other industries. This transformation has come alongside what many perceived as a threat to residential care: the implementation of the new community care policy.

Up to the end of 1970s it was local authorities that were the largest provider of residential care, but by the mid-1990s over 70 per cent were in private ownership. Throughout the 1980s a long-standing policy of closing large mental hospitals was speeded up. At the same time, the NHS began to reduce its provision for elderly people. It began to concentrate on acute care, and the view was taken that many elderly and disabled people who were formerly its responsibility should become the responsibility of social services departments because their needs were described as social rather than medical. However, the boundary between health and social care is not always clear. It was necessary for health and local authorities to work together in many circumstances and to include housing and voluntary agencies in their planning. The assessment of need became paramount, with resources being allocated according to eligibility criteria and within the strict financial boundaries set by national and local government. Thus the advent of community care was bound to have a significant effect on residential care – and it did.

'Community care' – so often taken to mean care at home – should mean care anywhere in the community, including residential homes. If a residential care home is not part of the community, it cannot be playing its role to the full. If isolation still exists, this compounds the view that residential care is only for those who do not fit within the mainstream of society and therefore has stigmatising effects for its consumers. Young people in children's homes are more often than not considered by the mere nature of being placed away from the parental home to be 'disturbed' or 'criminal'. Social services departments inadvertently promoted this perception by taking policy decisions in the 1980s and onwards that only 'difficult-to-place' children should be in children's homes, with an emphasis given to fostering. Whilst this may have been right for some children, for others who could no longer live in the parental home it meant inappropriate foster care placements time after time. Documentation from the National Association of Young People in Care (NAYPIC) showed clearly that many adolescents felt that offering an alternative family during the teenage years was highly inappropriate and sometimes insulting. Social work teaching encouraged the view that individual social workers had failed if their clients became subject to residential care. Employment in residential child care was seen by many simply as a stepping stone to other work in social services. The major charitable child care organisations, some by choice, others by lack of support from local authorities, turned away from residential child care to other forms of care for children. For these reasons, a service that had provided so much for some children itself began to accept, wrongly, the conviction that residential care was an unsuitable way of caring for children.

The law still required the provision of residential child care, but, for the reasons we have suggested, resources were not forthcoming and unit costs soared. Buildings were neglected, and it was easy to understand why children, when placed in a 'dump', would treat it as a 'dump'. Residential child care for some was and is unsuitable, but this persistent undermining of its strengths took its toll, and, from being at the forefront of residential services, morale plummeted and in certain cases standards with it.

There has also been a transformation in residential care for elderly people but in a different way from that in child care. Families find it increasingly difficult to look after a highly dependent parent due to economic pressures, changes in family structure and expectations about filial obligation. Older people are not prepared to be a 'burden' on their family and are much more readily prepared to consider a placement in a residential home. Radical changes in social security regulations in the early 1980s, which provided payments to individuals to fund living in private residential homes, led to an unprecedented increase in the provision of residential care for elderly people. An assessment of need by a professional was not always necessary, so the private sector boomed, with many small hotels becoming residential care homes. The result was that social security costs increased phenomenally and the Conservative government was forced to take steps to curb expenditure.

The Griffiths report and the Community Care legislation that followed gave the opportunity for major changes, and the responsibility for agreeing funding after an assessment was transferred to local authorities. Government demanded, however, that a significant percentage of the funding must be spent in the independent sector in order to promote competition in what had previously been a monoploy of local authority providers. However, problems with the new market soon emerged. Over-provision in some parts of the country, and a restriction on the amount that was paid by local authorities per resident, led to severe difficulties for providers and underfunded service users. Self-funding residents began to find that their own resources – including the family home – were soon disappearing, and media attention forced the government to increase the range of eligibility for funding. The concern of the various agencies to protect their own funding following the community care legislation became a major issue. Health Trusts were no longer willing to permit the use of hospital beds for long-term care, which they believed could be undertaken in a residential home where the costs would have to be met from social services budgets. Local authorities would not necessarily undertake the responsibility and 'bottlenecks' developed, with bed-blocking in acute medical services. In addition, increasing dependency of residents meant that the disparity between care in a nursing home and a residential care home became less obvious. A conviction that care in the community was always preferable has resulted in a situation whereby placement in a home has become a last resort and dependency so great that there is simply no alternative. In these ways, therefore, conflict and confusion have also come to characterise the provision of residential care for elderly people.

It is perhaps in services for people with learning disability that the most positive developments have taken place. Relatives have had a significant influence on the form of services available for this client group. Large institutions have disappeared, to be replaced by smaller units. Some agencies took the view that the provision of service should be centred around very small units, often consisting of no more than four residents with a minimum of staffing. Although some relatives are concerned that this makes too great a demand on the residents and renders them more vulnerable, there being also some doubts in relation to financial viability, there is no question that community care has pushed further positive changes that had begun to take place for this group of service users. In contrast to the developments in residential care for children and older people, a newly found confidence pervades the service, promoting a positive outlook for groups of people who could formerly only look forward to a sterile lifestyle, often involving menial tasks in large institutions.

In relation to people with mental disorders, considerable public concern has also been aroused about the decanting of thousands of people from large, old psychiatric hospitals. The policy decision taken, whilst morally admirable, has never been matched with resources, and, although large hospital wards were seen to be horrendous, they were at least able to provide minimal care and security for their inmates. Many service users had spent a considerable part of their life in such settings and found it difficult to cope in smaller units or living on their own. Homelessness for people with a mental illness became a common occurrence.

Thus, in all these forms of residential provision, the advent of the new community care has brought transformation – and all too often disillusion and confusion. There is now an urgent need for a reassessment of the role of residential institutions in community care. It would be difficult to promote residential care as the panacea for all people who find difficulty living in their own home, but there can be no doubt that, for a significant number, it provides an alternative to deprivation in a number of essential facets of life. It is ridiculous to seek to maintain that residential care can provide the same type of privacy and independence that may be available in one's own home. Note, however, that I say 'may be available', for we delude ourselves if we believe that, for example, an elderly, disabled and housebound person has much independence of choice. The Residential Forum, in its first publication, *A Standards Guide for Residential Care*, defined a home as:

> A place whose purpose includes the provision of residential accommodation, care and services for people who choose to live in a group or whose needs are best met through group care.

Group care will be suitable and acceptable for some but not for others. High-quality residential care can provide an alternative lifestyle, with the potential for gaining or regaining some opportunities, albeit whilst sacrificing others. It is an alternative choice that there is reason to believe will become more, rather than less, attractive to many people. Demography indicates that elderly people will live longer and form a greater percentage of the population. As I have suggested, the expectations of older people and their relatives about the possibility and desirability of very dependent elders being cared for by relatives at home are changing. Older people do not wish to be seen as a 'burden' on their family. There will always be people with learning disabilities who will only be able to function to the maximum of their abilities with support in residential accommodation. A similar position applies to many people with severe physical disability and chronic illness. A gradual recognition is taking place that people formerly looked after in mental hospitals on a long-term basis will require some sort of residential care. A complete rethink of how we look after children who are unable for whatever reason to live with their own family will need to be undertaken. Residential care will still be a better alternative, for some, than foster care and will need to be considered as a first rather than a last resort to end the outrage, for some teenagers, of persistent failed foster placements.

It would be naïve dogmatically to assert that all forms of residential care are here to stay, simply in defiance of those who find institutional care unsatisfactory. It would be more realistic and positive to say that good-quality residential care is here to stay. The mid-1990s have brought a surge of quality assurance systems, all to differing degrees enabling us to monitor and promote customer satisfaction. The development of national standards for residential care is an obvious course for government to take to ensure uniformity of approach, and much has recently been accomplished in this direction. All involved in the social care services see the value of regulation of the industry to ensure that people who are entrusted with other people's lives are appropriately qualified and licensed. No other profession dealing with people in such a personal way is willing to let untrained people take on the most complex and intimate tasks as is residential care. The days of full-time, college-based training for the majority of staff seem to have passed. Vocational, competence-based training in the workplace is more acceptable and financially viable for the majority of providers and is increasingly accessible. The restoration of full public confidence will depend on the service being regulated, and the introduction of a General Social Services Council will be paramount in ensuring that people have a license to practice and that such practice is monitored.

Perhaps most important of all is the restoration of the morale of staff who have constantly experienced criticism of the service in which they work and devaluation of their professional skills. They have endured financial and other forms of neglect for decades and have felt threatened by the lack of support given by those who should have been responsible for promoting residential care. Thus residential services have been racked with self-doubt because they have had to spend so much time looking over their shoulder and wondering what others might think. Service users need residential staff to be able to act in an appropriate way to provide support and care that is creative and allows for people to operate to the maximum of their ability in surroundings that are safe. In order to do so, staff must be confident in their own worth and that of the form of service they are providing. Many people will, in the coming years, rely on residential care, and there is a duty for all those involved to ensure that institutional care is perceived as a potential first choice and not as an undesirable last resort.

References

Residential Forum (1996) *A Standards Guide for Residential Care*. London, National Institute for Social Work.

INDEX